REAL SELF-CARE

life

REAL SELF-CARE

A TRANSFORMATIVE PROGRAM FOR REDEFINING WELLNESS

(CRYSTALS, CLEANSES, AND BUBBLE BATHS NOT INCLUDED)

POOJA LAKSHMIN, MD

PENGUIN LIFE

VIKING
An imprint of Penguin Random House LLC
penguinrandomhouse.com

A Penguin Life Book

Grateful acknowledgment is made for permission to reprint brief
excerpts from essays published in *The New York Times* that are featured
in this book. Pooja Lakshmin © 2022 The New York Times Company.

LIBRARY OF CONGRESS CATALOGING-IN-PUBLICATION DATA
Title: Real self-care : a transformative program for redefining
    wellness (crystals, cleanses, and bubble baths not included) /
    Pooja Lakshmin, MD.
Description. [New York, NY] : Penguin Life, [2023] |
    Includes bibliographical references.
Identifiers: LCCN 2022042721 | ISBN 9780593489727 (hardcover) |
    ISBN 9780593489734 (ebook)
Subjects: LCSH: Self-care, Health.
Classification: LCC RA776.95 .L335 2023 |
    DDC 613—dc23/eng/20221114
LC record available at https://lccn.loc.gov/2022042721

Printed in the United States of America
3rd Printing

Book design by Daniel Lagin

This book was written for every woman who wonders if she's got it all wrong, if she'll ever measure up, if she's asking for too much. I see you—I am you. Together, we will forge a better path, for ourselves and for the next generation.

For the master's tools will never dismantle the master's house. They may allow us temporarily to beat him at his own game, but they will never enable us to bring about genuine change.

AUDRE LORDE

Contents

Author's Note

You'll notice that I reference my patients in this book. Names and details have been changed in order to protect their privacy. In a couple instances, I have created composites out of an abundance of caution.

In this book you will find tools based on techniques that are commonly utilized in psychotherapy. *Real Self-Care* is meant to be a source of support and education. It is not a substitute for seeking professional help and treatment. At the end of the book, I have included resources for finding a mental health professional.

I've created a space for folks who are practicing *Real Self-Care* to come together. Join me and my colleagues at Gemma: the physician-led women's mental health community that centers equity and impact www.gemmawomen.com.

Introduction

You may have noticed that lately it's nearly impossible to go even a couple of days without coming across the term *self-care*. A phrase that encompasses any number of lifestyle choices or products—from juice cleanses to yoga workshops to luxury bamboo sheets—"self-care" has exploded in our collective consciousness as a panacea for practically all women's problems.

As a physician specializing in women's mental health, I find this cultural embrace of self-care incomplete at best, and manipulative at worst. Wellness dogma says that a fix for your troubles is as simple as buying a new day planner or signing up for a meditation class. And according to this philosophy, when you don't find time for these "solutions," it's your fault for not keeping up with one more task on your to-do list. In my clinical practice, where I take care of women suffering from burnout, demoralization, depression, and anxiety, I have seen countless patients come in and say some version of: "Dr. Lakshmin, I feel like crap. Everything feels like a chore, I'm constantly on edge—and I feel like it's my fault because I'm not doing self-care!"

It's not their fault and it's not yours.

In reality, the game is rigged.

By focusing on *faux* self-care—what I call the products and solutions marketed to us as remedies—we've conceptualized self-care all wrong. Faux self-care is largely full of empty calories and devoid of substance. It keeps us looking outward—comparing ourselves with others or striving for a certain type of perfection—which means it's incapable of truly nourishing us in the long run.

It's understandable that we turn to faux self-care and wellness to solve our problems—after all, it's everywhere we look! And as you'll see in the introduction here, I've done it too. When we're feeling exhausted and in despair and we see an ad for the latest juice cleanse promising extraordinary results, *of course* our ears perk up. So please, let me be clear, I don't mean to shame anyone who takes solace in wellness as a respite from their hectic lives—that's not the point of this book. Instead, I'm here to share that not only is the helplessness that we feel when it comes to taking care of ourselves *not our fault*, there is also a better way to do it, from the inside out, and that's precisely what I am going to teach you.

In this book you'll learn how to carve out a meaningful path forward. Real self-care, as you'll see, is not a one-stop shop like a fancy spa retreat or a journaling app; it's an internal process that involves making difficult decisions that will pay off tenfold in the long run as a life built around the relationships and activities that matter most to you. My goal is to teach you the difference between the two not only by lifting the veil on commodified faux self-care but also by transforming your understanding of what a real practice of caring for yourself could look like and showing you that it's possible. I'll share practical tools and tangible strategies for how you can make wellness your own—making positive changes in your own life and then expanding that knowledge outward, to impact the people and systems around you. As I'll teach you in this book, real self-care not only impacts us as individuals—it also has a cascade effect in our relationships, communities and workplaces, and society at large. It is what we need not only to buffer ourselves but also to change the systems that are not serving us as women.

In short, there is a better way.

WHY LISTEN TO ME?

I've spent the better part of the past decade working as a psychiatrist specializing in women's mental health, in addition to twelve years of education to become a physician and a psychiatrist. In my clinical work I've spent thousands of hours taking care of women struggling with burnout, despair, depression, and anxiety. In addition to treating patients and my academic endeavors, I've poured myself into gender and social justice advocacy.

But perhaps more important than my professional accolades is for you to know that I've been there—*right where you are.* I've believed that if I followed the recipe of fancy schools, a prestigious career, and marriage, my feelings would catch up and I'd feel content and fulfilled. I've suffered from burnout, hopeless-ness, and even clinical depression and anxiety. I've taken medi-cation and been in psychotherapy. I've been through loss, hardship, and trauma. And I've made a number of mistakes on my journey (some of which are detailed in this book).

A decade ago, while in my late twenties, after spending much of my life up until that point in school to become a physician, I made a drastic decision. To the shock and horror of my family and friends, in the course of a year I blew up my marriage, moved into a wellness commune in San Francisco, and dropped out of my highly competitive psychiatry residency training program. And not just any commune, but one that practiced and taught orgasmic meditation.

Convinced I had found the Answer to life's problems, I spent nearly two years with this group—living in their intentional community, working for their wellness start-up, and spreading their message with fervor. The group itself was organized like a matriarchy, in which women held and wielded the power. To say this appealed to me was putting it lightly; I was a former wom-en's studies major but had grown up in a patriarchal South Asian culture and had just gone through a male-dominated academic medical system.

In the introductory class for the group, co-led by an ob-gyn, the group's leader explained that the reason women felt unsat-isfied was because Western culture had indoctrinated us to disconnect from our bodies, and because of that, we never learned to fully live in our power. They offered up orgasmic meditation as a female-focused practice that was akin to sensate focus therapy—it allowed you to drop away from all the noise and chatter in your brain and connect with your body, and in turn, with yourself. Within a week of that first class, I dove in. It was the first time in my life that I saw women openly asking for what they wanted and getting it. It felt like the one wellness practice—the one feminist utopia—that could fix all of my problems. I spent nearly two years deeply immersed in this group's world of spiritual practice and Eastern wellness modalities.

How did a type A, perfectionistic physician find herself in a group focusing on female orgasm? In hindsight, I realize I had been simultaneously searching desperately to find myself in new and exciting places while also attempting to lose myself. I was disillusioned with mainstream medicine and psychiatry, which, at the time, I viewed as irredeemably flawed and betraying the people it proposed to help. As a trainee, I experienced the death of a patient, which crushed me. I started to question what was being taught—I didn't get much guidance in medical school or residency on what to do when your patient can't pay for health insurance or when she has lost childcare for the third time in two months and is being fired from her job. Instead, I was taught to prescribe medications or provide psychotherapy for issues that were clearly systemic. While there is certainly a great need for both of these medical interventions, the lack of attention to the inhumanity of our social policies left me feeling powerless—just like my patients. Personally, I was burned out and teetering on depression, and I felt like my own attempts to get professional help were lacking (despite being a physician myself!). It was in this state—angry and feeling betrayed by our medical system—that I left to find answers in the most unlikely of places.

To me, the group I joined was changing the world—breaking stigmas and taboos about women's sexual well-being and fighting loudly for the empowerment of people who are often dismissed by the medical establishment. I met the neuroscientists at the Rutgers fMRI orgasm lab, one of only two labs in the world that studied female orgasm through brain imaging technology. I studied what happens in the brain during female orgasm. It was a period of both personal and academic exploration.

During this time, I became aware of many critics of the group, yet I didn't have tolerance for them. From my perspective, I was there fully of my own volition, and I looked with pity upon those who couldn't see how singular this group and its mission were. At the time, I believed in their particular brand of wellness dogma and spirituality—a combination of new age teaching and Silicon Valley–espoused libertarianism. Coincidentally, the dogma fit perfectly with my Hindu upbringing, which leaned heavily on magical thinking, mythology, and gurus.

Unfortunately, what I didn't realize, and what those who cared about me did, was that as a physician, I offered something invaluable: legitimacy. During the time I was with the group, from 2012 to 2013, I was treated with kid gloves, kept at arm's length from the inner workings of the higher-ups. At the time, I thought that distance was in place because I was not spiritually actualized enough to be in the inner circle. It was many years later, in

2018 after the news broke about an FBI investigation into this group, that I found out how dark the story had become and I put together the pieces of why I was always shooed away.

I left the group after a little less than two years. As they were reaching new levels of success and opening wellness centers all over the world, I began to notice inconsistencies in their dogma. I wanted to finish my residency training, and I was starting to understand that one wellness practice could not fix all of my problems.

It wasn't until I left and started doing my own healing that I recognized how much my time in the group had warped my thinking. I struggled to make sense of what had happened. I fell into a deep depression and wondered if I could keep living. I no longer had the group, and in the process of joining it I had torched my old life.

I had to rebuild my life, and myself, largely from scratch.

My parents let me crash at their place, rent-free. I turned thirty in my old childhood bedroom, wrung out and bingeing reruns of *Law & Order: Special Victims Unit*, texting with the few close friends who stuck with me. I was fortunate to have mental health professionals to turn to who helped me work through my experiences and make meaning of them. Others who left the group didn't have that luxury and suffered much more than I did. And I had to grapple with the knowledge that I helped legitimize this group—a cult—as a physician and a professional who spoke publicly on their behalf while I was deeply entrenched in their philosophy.

It was understandable—like many of you, I dove into a wellness practice because the thought had not occurred to me that the solutions needed to come from inside myself. While the practice of orgasmic meditation had helped me personally, I had been seduced by the fantasy that an external solution—this shiny wellness practice—could fix all of the problems in my life.

Instead, I learned the hard way that self-care is an inside job.

Going on to face the real world by returning to my medical training was both the hardest thing I've done *and* the thing that's given me the most strength. In many ways, it was leaving the cult, not joining it, that has made me the person I am now. I learned to set boundaries, came to understand my values, and ultimately found my voice and started speaking up for myself—separate from my family, the medical system, and the cult. In short, I learned how to practice *real* self-care.

In the decade since then, I've come to understand that real self-care is not only a more authentic and sustainable solution—it's also self-determined. It involves the internal process of setting boundaries, learning to treat yourself with compassion, making choices that bring you closer to yourself, and living a life aligned with your values. It's hard work, but not only can it be achieved, it can be maintained internally, unlike an off-the-shelf product or the lessons of a self-help guru. And, as you'll come to understand in this book, it has the potential to shift our relationships, our workplace culture, and even our social systems, thus impacting the collective injustices that are the root of women's problems.

I ultimately graduated psychiatry residency and joined the

faculty at George Washington University School of Medicine, then went on to start my own private practice focused on women's mental health. You won't be surprised to learn that when my patients began coming in talking about self-care and wellness solutions like vaginal jade eggs and turmeric face masks, I was worried. On one hand, I understood that my patients, who were at their wit's end from demanding family lives and nonstop careers, were understandably looking to these solutions for a bit of solace. Yet I had tried extreme wellness and I knew the dangers of getting caught up in the self-care industrial complex. Now I not only had the credentials and the professional expertise to set the record straight, I also had this profound personal experience of what happens when wellness goes very wrong. And even more than that, I knew there was an alternative that was self-driven and sourced from the inside.

So, I did what any reasonable geriatric millennial would do—I started a blog and an Instagram account. Soon after, in 2018, I published an essay for *Doximity*—"We Don't Need Self-Care; We Need Boundaries." Aimed at an audience of women physicians, the piece was an attempt to shed light on the problematic nature of self-care as a solution for health-care worker burnout. Like in many industries, hospitals and medical groups were offering up "resilience training" as a solution to the burnout epidemic in clinicians. But despite these perks, there was no mention of paid time off, childcare subsidies, or real policy changes to support workers. In the weeks after the publication of my essay, I received message after message from women across the country telling me they felt like I was describing their exact plight. Subsequently, in 2019, *The New York Times* asked me to adapt the essay to speak more broadly to a nonmedical audience, and I went on to become a regular contributor, writing about gender justice, women's mental health, and the societal structures that prevent women from being able to build emotional well-being.

From all these seeds grew the book you hold in your hands.

Before we go any further, I want to be clear with you. For a long time, I hesitated in writing about this topic and joining the self-help field. I am not writing as your guru. If it's someone else's answer, it can never be your solution. Whether it's a full-fledged cult, a diet, or the latest fitness program, the answer to your problems is never going to be someone else telling you what to do, myself included. As you'll understand as you dive into this book, the answers can only come from inside you. As you read along, you will notice that I don't prescribe a lot of rules to follow, but rather encourage you to ask tough questions and make hard decisions. This is deliberate—from what I know, personally and professionally, real self-care has to come from within you. What I'm providing is a guide to hold space for your own self-reflection, and productive questions to ask yourself, so that ultimately, you can create your own path for meaningful and long-term real self-care.

WHAT YOU'LL LEARN HERE

In this book, I'm going to teach you why self-care as we've conceptualized it is all wrong, and arm you with the crucial tools you need to do the radical work of taking real care of yourself. This work isn't about fixing yourself—in fact, it's high time we stop telling women they need to be fixed. Instead, I will teach you how to care for yourself from the inside and, in turn, create a cascade effect that influences your family, your relationships, and even your workplace. Real self-care is revolutionary precisely because it has the power to change the root cause of our problems—the systems.

Some of this work will be challenging for you—as women we are taught that caring for ourselves is a selfish act. We learn early in life that we should be putting our energy into caring for others (as daughters, partners, mothers, etc.). I am giving you permission to hold space for yourself as you read this book. Do not shy away from taking this time to learn how to look after your own well-being. What you learn here may go against what you've been taught, but it is not self-indulgent—*it's necessary.*

That being said, this book is predicated on the notion of dispelling the myth and the *burden* that you can have it all, so don't worry—I'm not going to give you another set of ideals or practices to fail at. Instead, I will invite you to take a close look at how you spend your time and how you talk to yourself, so you can make clear decisions about aligning your behaviors with what matters most to you.

In Part I, I'm going to show you the systemic problematic nature of what I call *faux* self-care. You'll understand why faux self-care is an empty promise that skips the critical self-driven process of developing boundaries and identifying what truly nourishes us. We will examine the way our patriarchal society has saddled women with the mental load, leaving us burned out, disconnected, and primed to practice faux self-care as an individual solution to a societal problem. We'll also dive into the three main ways women are understandably seduced into faux self-care as a coping mechanism: escape, achievement, and optimization. Finally, you will get a bird's-eye view of how the individual practice of real self-care has the power to impact the people and systems in your life. I'll describe cases from my clinical practice, explain the latest scientific research on well-being, and share personal stories from my own life experiences as a woman who has grappled, often in messy and unproductive ways, with how to implement real self-care.

In Part II of the book, we will roll up our sleeves and get to work. I'll teach you about eudaimonic well-being and why real self-care is grounded in this psychological concept. Then I'll share with you my framework—the Four Principles of Real Self-Care:

1. Set boundaries with others.
2. Change how you talk to yourself.
3. Bring in what matters most *to you*.
4. This is power—use it for good.

In these chapters you will also find actionable tools and exercises to help you start putting these principles into practice right away. I recommend reading the chapters in the order I've laid them out, so you have a full understanding of how they build on each other. Then, as you're implementing your real self-care practice in your life, feel free shift back and forth. The end of this book contains an appendix of exercises so you can easily reference these tools in the future.

LET'S GET STARTED

This book is my letter to every woman out there who has flirted with hopping in the car and running away from it all. To the women who are so bogged down in the mess of things that they don't even stop to imagine running away from it all. I want this to be a powerful resource for you and the scores of women, like you and me, who feel let down by the gratitude lists, the meditation apps, and the essential oils. It's not just that the status quo is broken; it's that the extent of the brokenness demands massive and radical change—*and that change starts inside all of us.*

You'll come away from *Real Self-Care* armed with clarity on how to develop practices that are truly nourishing—and transforming. In the end, you'll understand that real self-care is not a noun—it's a *verb*. And while it won't be as easy as buying that crystal-infused water bottle, it sure works a lot better.

A Word on Identity, Privilege, and Systems of Oppression

'm writing this book from the perspective of a cis-hetero second-generation South Asian American woman. I was raised in southeast Pennsylvania by my immigrant parents—a physician father and a homemaker mother. Growing up, I spent a good deal of time in Bangalore, India, where my parents and my extended family are originally from, which has greatly informed my view of the world.

You'll notice I use the word *women* throughout the book. The definition I am using is borrowed from Silvia Federici,[1] who, when asked to define the term *women*, has said: "To me it has always been mostly in terms of a political category." I use the word *women* inclusively to mean all people who suffer under the oppressive conditions that have typically been associated with the female sex, which includes queer folks, trans and nonbinary people, and intersex and agender people.

My clinical practice is focused on people who identify as women, many of whom have children but not all. In a country without mandatory paid family leave and with astronomical childcare costs, parenthood can be an existential tipping point for women. But it is important to note that it's not just mothers who suffer from this overburdening—it's anyone who has been conditioned to put the needs and preferences of others ahead of themselves.

It's also important to note that systems of power affect individuals differently—those who have privileges like financial resources, family support, or lighter skin will have an easier time enacting change in their lives, while those who are the most marginalized may have to work harder to achieve the same outward results. Black and Indigenous women, trans and queer women, women living in poverty, and those who hold multiple vulnerable identities are more often than not the ones who are the most encumbered. This is precisely why we must shift away from a commodified version of wellness, which continues to uphold and perpetuate inequitable systems of power. As you'll learn throughout this book, real self-care is a radical and necessary practice for people of marginalized identities—it's a strategy for taking power away from predatory systems, bringing it back into yourself, and ultimately enacting change. Self-help traditionally does not acknowledge the systemic barriers that women and people from marginalized groups face. I wanted to change that: throughout the book, you'll see that I reference systems of oppression—racism, toxic capitalism, sexism, and ableism. While it's not meant as an exhaustive list, the tools you'll learn here will bring to light how these systems become internalized. At the end of the book, I have included resources to find mental health professionals who specialize in working with members of minority communities.

REAL SELF-CARE

PART I

THE TYRANNY OF FAUX SELF-CARE

Chapter 1

EMPTY CALORIES

FAUX SELF-CARE
HASN'T SAVED US

––––––

Revolutions that last don't happen from the top down.
They happen from the bottom up.

GLORIA STEINEM

My patient Erin, thirty-eight, a mom of three school-age kids, wanted to pull her hair out whenever she heard the term *self-care*. She was up before 5:00 a.m. most mornings, responding to emails, getting the kids ready for school, and then rushing into the office for a ten-hour day. In the evenings, she'd pick up the kids and prep dinner before helping with homework and bedtime routines. Around 9:30 p.m., she would open up her laptop again for another two hours of work.

"Just tell me, when in this chaos am I supposed to find time for self-care?" she lamented. "I don't need a two-hundred-dollar massage, though it sure would be nice. I need more than five hours of sleep a night."

Whenever Erin found a couple of minutes to look into doing

something for herself, the advice she found felt painfully condescending: "learn how to meditate" or "make a gratitude list." Instead of giving her a sense of relief, these recommendations just made Erin feel bad. "If everyone else seems to feel better with a bubble bath and a glass of wine, what's wrong with me that I can't get it together to make that happen?"

Then there was Hina, twenty-nine, who was struggling to achieve that elusive work-life balance. In her pursuit, she found herself diving headfirst into optimization and productivity strategies. She was always the first in her group of friends to try out the new meal delivery service and was fortunate to be able to outsource household tasks from time to time. Her focus on productivity was theoretically in service of finding time to do self-care, yet Hina could never quite pour the time she gained back into herself. When she did grab an extra hour for herself, she felt irritated by the leftover dishes in the sink and plagued by guilt for not spending more time at work.

These stories are common in my clinical practice, where, as a psychiatrist, I specialize in women's mental health. I see women of all backgrounds and ages—single and partnered, mothers and those who are child-free. Some of these women are coping with depression or anxiety, but many are just struggling to figure out how to take care of themselves in the midst of incredibly busy and hectic lives—and that was before a pandemic raised our stress and anxiety levels to epic proportions. The commonality among all of these women is clear, though—they're struggling, and what they're doing to find relief isn't working.

THE BROKEN PROMISES OF FAUX SELF-CARE

In the past few years, I've noticed something curious happening. For women, the cultural obsession with self-care has not only failed to provide solace, it has also added more guilt and pressure. A common refrain I hear in my practice is "I'm burned out, I just can't do it anymore, *and* I feel like it's my fault because I *should* be taking care of myself." Self-care ends up being another burden, another thing on the to-do list for women to feel bad about because they aren't doing it right. I call this the *tyranny of self-care.*

My patients feel beaten down and confused, and so do I. And, taking it a step further, many of us also understandably feel insulted and resentful that not only do we not have time for these "strategies," but even when we do them, they don't provide the relief that is advertised. Or on the occasions when they do work, the relief doesn't last long. We are right to recognize that it's ridiculous that the solution we are sold to the unrelenting demands of being a woman in the twenty-first century is a twenty-dollar bath bomb. Our culture has taken wellness and foisted it on the individual—where it can be bought, measured, and held up as personal success—instead of investing in making our social systems healthy.

Personally, I also know the allure of these supposed fixes all too well—I shared in the introduction about my wellness-cult deep dive. But even before that dramatic decision, in my early twenties I turned to yoga as a fix for being a burned-out medical student. It certainly helped at first—my weekly yoga class was a much-needed break from memorizing the Krebs cycle, and I felt stronger in my body. But like a pattern I observe with many of my patients, I brought the same perfectionistic mindset to yoga that I took to medical school. When I couldn't keep up with the rigid yoga schedule I had outlined, I quickly chalked myself up as a failure.

There was also that time I subscribed to *Real Simple* magazine, convinced that if I gained mastery over my out-of-control closet, a feeling of inner contentment would closely follow. (I'm only slightly embarrassed to report that there's still a pile of *Real Simple* magazines collecting dust at the bottom of my closet.)

The data backs up the fact that commodified wellness is not working. American women not only report higher stress levels than men but also feel they are not doing a good job of managing it.[1] A 2018 Canadian study of more than two thousand workers found that women reported higher levels of burnout compared to men.[2] A systematic review from the University of Cambridge conducted across Europe and North America found that women are nearly twice as likely to suffer from anxiety as men, and there is a similar discrepancy when it comes to depression.[3] One in five women ages forty to fifty-nine and nearly one in four women sixty and over were prescribed antidepressant medications in the United States, according to data from 2015 to 2018. For women ages eighteen to thirty-nine, the number was closer to one in ten.[4]

Yet, curiously, search Instagram and you'll find more than

sixty million posts tagged with #SelfCare. They run the gamut from beachside yoga to triumphant mommy blogs to "curative" smoothie recipes. If we use social media as our guide, self-care appears to be . . . anything that looks good in a photo?

As I mentioned earlier, this is faux self-care—the wellness behaviors and practices that are commonly sold as a remedy for women's problems. In many cases, faux self-care is just a sugar high, serving as an escape from the realities of daily life and moving us further away from our true selves. Faux self-care is also big business. A report from the Global Wellness Institute found that the global wellness industry, which is targeted at women in particular, was worth $4.4 trillion in 2020.[5] While products like crystal-infused water bottles and vagus nerve pillow sprays might elicit a temporary sense of calm (putting aside the fact that they are too pricey for most American women), they do nothing to change the social systems that have us craving relief in the first place—so the cycle of consumerism continues unabated. Faux self-care is *faux* because when used alone, without the critical internal work we will discuss in this book, it does nothing to change our larger systems.

A NOTE ON SOCIAL MEDIA INFLUENCERS

If you're like me, you might find yourself browsing Instagram or other social media apps and wondering how on earth women find the time to have a perfectly curated home, gorgeous children, and on-point hair and makeup. It's so easy to look at influencer accounts and feel like "Wow, they're doing it, it looks so easy—why do I feel like a mess?" And when they share about a wellness product, it's understandable to be curious and think, "Maybe this product is the perfect solution to my problems!"

When you find yourself feeling this way, I encourage you to take a beat. Because influencers are on our phones, and our phones are with us all the time, it's easy to feel artificially close to them. But remember that social media is a highlight reel. When you see an influencer touting a wellness product, look to see if this person is being paid to promote it (i.e., it's a sponsored post). Influencers have the opportunity to play a role in shifting the dynamic in commodified wellness, and while some do speak up for social and policy change, not all are discerning about the wellness industry. Pay attention to which issues they speak up on, how they disclose the behind-the-scenes of their own lives, and what sort of vetting they do when promoting wellness products. If you notice that an influencer is not engaging in transparency or due diligence, reflect on if following them is making you feel better or worse about yourself. While there is a growing cohort of influencers who are making informed and conscious decisions about how they engage with the wellness industry, the social media space is still very much the wild,

wild west. As a prime target of the wellness industry, you are exerting agency—and thus power—when you apply a critical lens to how you engage with influencers and social media marketing.

SELF-CARE: IT HASN'T ALWAYS BEEN TYRANNICAL

Because self-care is everywhere you turn these days—whether it's social media, podcasts, or our text threads with friends—it's tempting to believe that it's a uniquely twenty-first-century concept. The reality is that the 2020s version of self-care has come a long way from its beginnings. It turns out that self-care has two major lines of origin: health care and social justice. Self-care's origin story is fascinating and helpful for understanding why faux self-care occupies the large and expanding space it does today. Inside its origin story, we can also find some clues on how to reclaim self-care as our own.

Seventy-some years ago, in the 1950s, psychiatrists used the term *self-care* to describe the ways in which institutionalized patients could assert independence by taking charge of their diets and engaging in exercise while in the hospital. By the 1960s, nursing and medical professionals talked about their own need for self-care in response to compassion fatigue and secondary trauma. Fast-forward to the 1970s and self-care moved from the medical community to activist circles, with the Black Panther

Party promoting self-care as a means for Black Americans to preserve their humanity in the face of systemic racism. It was Black women who actualized the concept into public discourse. Audre Lorde defined self-care as a powerful act to reclaim space within a society that demanded minorities and oppressed groups stay small or invisible. As she wrote in her 1988 book, *A Burst of Light*, "Caring for myself is not self-indulgence, it is self-preservation, and that is an act of political warfare."[6] As we'll discuss in Chapter 3, real self-care is built on this very notion and, when implemented authentically, has the potential to change our broken system.

By the 1990s, as the economics of health care in the US were shifting, health-care professionals began encouraging patients with chronic medical conditions like diabetes and high blood pressure to take primary responsibility for their health as opposed to being passive recipients of care.[7] Researchers found that for those living with chronic illnesses, self-care in the form of exercise, healthy diet, stress management, and other lifestyle interventions was associated with better health outcomes.[8]

Self-care as the so-called cure that we now know it as evolved when the world became more hyperconnected. As we transitioned to smartphones, a twenty-four-hour news cycle, and a plethora of ways to keep up with family, friends, and complete strangers via social media, we also saw a parallel need for a balm from that stimulation overload. Self-care was no longer relegated to the realm of health, nor was it about standing up against oppressive systems. Instead, it morphed into a release valve, designed to bring you a momentary sense that things are all right. By the 2010s, the term *self-care* had exploded on social media and in the daily fabric of women's lives. The more out of control and dysfunctional our social structures became, the more our social media feeds were filled with glossy images of women seemingly living their best lives in picturesque locations. (Interestingly, Google searches for *self-care* peaked in November 2016, following election night in the United States.)[9]

As a psychiatrist, I'm understandably interested in the connection between the explosion of faux self-care and the status of mental health treatment. While not everyone who engages with faux self-care needs professional mental health services, the symptoms of a major depressive disorder or a clinical anxiety disorder have quite a bit of overlap with those of burnout and chronic stress. But mental health treatment (like seeing a psychotherapist or a psychiatrist) is financially costly and typically not covered by insurance, and so remains inaccessible to many. It also takes time. The work of psychotherapy is not instantaneous—it can take months to see some progress (or to even get off a waiting list to be seen!). Similarly, trying to find the right medication can also take time. On the other hand, the seemingly easy and shiny solutions of faux self-care are, well, so much more simple and sexy. Why fight with your insurance company when you can buy a vitamin pack that your favorite influencer recommends, and it will be delivered to your door the next day?

So we can't talk about faux self-care without talking about mental health treatment. We also can't talk about any of this without acknowledging there is a huge gap in access to affordable mental health services. There are several parts to the interplay between mental health and wellness solutions—first, a lack of education and awareness for many women about what constitutes a clinical mental health condition. Then, there's the stigma that still exists around seeing a therapist or a psychiatrist. Finally, once you've crossed all of those not-insignificant hurdles, there is the lack of insurance coverage, and the fact that finding access to a good therapist and psychiatrist is still only possible for the most privileged in our society. It's in this context, where actual treatment for mental health conditions is inaccessible for the vast majority of folks, that our culture serves us faux self-care as a quick fix and as a poor substitute for professional help. I don't mean to shame anyone here—in fact, when you are clinically depressed or anxious, finding a therapist and calling up your insurance company is even more difficult. It's no wonder that we are vulnerable to the slick marketing of faux self-care.

The time has come for self-care to evolve again, to take on a new definition. And that definition requires looking deeper, turning inward, and developing a reliable internal method for yourself—not one that has been prescribed for you by a wellness company or an influencer, but instead a solution that comes from you.

> ## HOW TO KNOW WHEN IT'S TIME TO SEEK PROFESSIONAL HELP
>
> As a physician, it's important to me to point out that there is a difference between treatment for a mental health condition—like major depressive disorder—and wellness activities. It's crucial not to mistake faux self-care (or, for that matter, real self-care) as a treatment for a medical condition. Throughout the rest of the book, I will be pointing out key areas to take note of, how to tell the difference between a clinical condition and something that can be helped by real self-care, as well as indicators for when to think about seeking professional help. At the end of the book, I have included resources for finding a mental health professional.

FAUX SELF-CARE VERSUS REAL SELF-CARE

To illustrate the difference between faux self-care and real self-care, I offer the example of my patient Shelby. Shelby, a thirty-two-year-old married white woman, first came to see me for help managing her depression, which had long been under control with the help of psychotherapy and medication. During her time in treatment with me, she had her first baby. Shelby considered herself someone who had her act together. She had always been on top of her mental health, getting treatment for her depression in her early twenties, and had risen in the ranks of her career at a large ad agency. Shelby loved her job, and she loved getting things done. She had a healthy relationship with her husband, Mark, who had been her college sweetheart. When they decided to start trying for their first child together, they spent a good deal of time examining the various responsibilities they would each be in charge of and committed to an equal division of labor in the home. Together Shelby and Mark discussed all the different scenarios of how their finances would work and how much time she'd take off work because she was the primary breadwinner.

Shelby's main self-care strategy prior to having her daughter was exercise—she loved to run and also had an elliptical machine. She found that in addition to therapy and medication, daily exercise was incredibly important for her mental health and the health of her relationship.

Shelby went into labor a couple of weeks before her due date, and her daughter, Felicity, was born prematurely. Because Felicity was born early, her suck reflex was not fully mature, and she had trouble latching on to the nipple during breastfeeding. Shelby, ever the problem solver and the one to "get it done," set out to fix the issue. She took Felicity to a specialist to fix her tongue-tie, and diligently followed the pediatrician's recommendation to *triple feed*, meaning that every feed involved three steps: putting Felicity to the breast for a period of time, pumping milk in order to keep her supply up, and then giving Felicity high-calorie formula to encourage her to gain weight.

Despite this, Felicity was not putting on weight as she should and was falling off the growth curve. Each feed was a knockdown, drag-out fight, as Felicity did not like breastfeeding. Each session typically ended in tears (for both Felicity and Shelby). During this time, Shelby, in her sleep-deprived state, tried to find comfort in her typical self-care activity of exercise. She couldn't run postpartum, so she used her elliptical. However, she had very little time to work out and when she did, she became upset that her body couldn't perform like it used to. She went to a mommy and me postpartum stress class, but that only added more pressure as she compared Felicity's development to all the other infants'. The harder she pushed at some of these self-care solutions (which had worked for her in the past), the more disconnected Shelby felt from herself and from her family.

One day in a therapy session with me, Shelby described a new feeling that she was just starting to understand. During the triple feeds, after Felicity and Shelby would have their knockdown fight at the breast, Shelby would hand her daughter off to her husband to bottle-feed, burp, and soothe while Shelby pumped breast milk. In those moments, Shelby found herself looking at her husband with a combination of envy and resentment. He got to spend quality time experiencing the best of their cute little daughter—meanwhile, as a mother, she was forced into the misery of trying to make something work that was clearly not working. Shelby also realized that she was starting to develop negative feelings toward her daughter—she resented Felicity for not getting with the program and breastfeeding like she was supposed to. And, in the same breath, she realized that if she wanted to be the mother she hoped that she'd become, she would have to let go of breastfeeding. Once Shelby made this tough decision, she noticed that she started to feel more like herself. She was sleeping a little more and felt more comfortable in her body. She found herself going on short runs again, without having to force herself. She felt more relaxed in group settings with other mothers.

In his bestselling book *Effortless*, author and leadership expert Greg McKeown elucidates an important point about decision-making—the difference between methods and principles. He writes: "A method may be useful once, to solve one specific type of problem. Principles, however, can be applied broadly and repeatedly."[10] Faux self-care is a *method*—in the moment, going for a run might improve your mood, but it does nothing to change the circumstances in your life that led you to feel drained, energy-less, or down. On the other hand, the work of real self-care is about going deeper and identifying the core *principles* to guide decision-making. When you apply these principles to your life, you don't just feel relief in the moment, you design a system of living that prevents the problems from coming up in the first place. In other words, applying a methodology of faux self-care is reactive, whereas practicing real self-care is proactive. To bring it back to Shelby—exercise and the postpartum group were methods that on the surface seemed helpful, but in this new phase of life, they weren't nourishing her anymore.

By deciding to stop breastfeeding, Shelby was turning to the principles of real self-care. She set boundaries (coming from a large family based locally, she had many relatives who loved to give unsolicited advice about feeding the baby); developed compassion for herself (by recognizing that resentment was building between her and her daughter, and her and her husband); identified her values (in prioritizing her relationships with her daughter and her husband); and asserted power (by using her agency to make a hard choice). Her particular method for real self-care as a new mother was to let go of breastfeeding and accept a new direction that prioritized her relationships.

To be clear, it's not that exercise or the support group were bad solutions (in fact, psychiatrists often recommend movement as an evidence-based strategy to mitigate mild depression). The issue was that exercise was causing psychological stress because Shelby was comparing her performance to her prepregnancy state. Similarly, in the postpartum group sessions, she was preoccupied with her baby's performance. Once she practiced real self-care and reworked her feeding plan for Felicity, Shelby found she was able to return to her workouts in a healthier fashion, and she was able to be compassionate toward herself in her moms' group.

As we move through the book, you will understand how your own *methods* of real self-care will differ based on your particular situation. But the *principles* are remarkably consistent. If you start implementing these principles in your life (and you don't even need to do it perfectly—you just need to start), then you'll find that your unique methods for real self-care become clear to you.

BUT WHAT IF I REALLY LIKE THE WELLNESS STUFF?

Shelby's story brings us to an important caveat. I know that some of you might enjoy and look forward to wellness practices—like yoga, meditation, or energy work. I'm not here to shame any of you who like to turn to wellness activities. In fact, in the years since I left the cult, I've been known to indulge in a Reiki session or two, even while writing this book! This might sound confusing to you, because the premise of the solution I'm proposing is seemingly counter to commodified wellness and so-called *woo-woo* practices. Hear me out—one person's yoga class can be profoundly nourishing, while another person's yoga class can simply be an avoidance strategy or an escape. Like we just discussed, there are an infinite number of *methods* you can use to take care of yourself—my goal here is to offer you the guiding *principles* that you can implement to uncover your own unique methods. *Real self-care is not a noun, it's a verb.* So it's possible for the work of real self-care (boundary setting, self-compassion, and getting clear on values) to point you in the direction of a wellness activity. For example, if you have a hard conversation with your partner about needing space in your week for your yoga class and go on to treat yourself kindly during that yoga class and reflect explicitly about how a yoga practice is in alignment with your values, this is real self-care! The internal work that gets you to the yoga class is the bit that carries forth sustainably and reliably—perhaps in some seasons of your life the method will be yoga, and in other seasons the method will be different. The internal process—real self-care—is timeless.

FAUX SELF-CARE VERSUS REAL SELF-CARE

When you first start out, it can be a little tricky to differentiate between faux self-care and real self-care. The following chart can help you spot the difference.

Faux Self-Care	Real Self-Care
Prescribed from outside	Originates within you
A noun, typically describing an activity or a product	A verb, describing an invisible, internal decision-making process
Common examples: a yoga class, a meditation app, or a fancy face cream	The internal process that goes on for you before you make the choice to attend the yoga class, listen to the meditation app, or put on the fancy face cream
Maintains status quo in your relationship or family, and does nothing to change larger systems	Allows you to get your needs met in your relationships, and can effect change in your family, workplace, and larger systems
Often leaves you feeling further away from yourself	Brings you closer to yourself and what's most important to you

Typically comes with feelings of guilt (either for never getting to it, or while you are engaging in it because you are neglecting other responsibilities)	Requires learning to cope with feelings of guilt as part of the process
Allows you to avoid or brush aside emotional costs or risks	Comes with a short-term emotional cost, in order to reap longer-term emotional gains

Now that you're getting a better sense of the difference between real self-care and faux self-care, consider the following questions:

- What types of faux self-care have you tried?
- When do you find yourself most likely to turn to faux self-care?
- What aspect of faux self-care has you feeling the most disappointed?
- Have there been certain activities or wellness practices that have helped you?
- Are there certain feelings or thoughts about yourself that these activities elicit?
- In order to integrate these helpful wellness activities into your life, have you noticed changes in how you talk to yourself or how you navigate your relationships? If so, what changes have you noticed?

As you move through the rest of the book, come back to these questions to distinguish for yourself which activities fall into the faux self-care category and which are aligned with real self-care. Over time, asking yourself these questions will feel second nature.

Chapter 2

WHY IT'S HARD TO
RESIST THE SEDUCTION

THE WAYS WE TURN
TO FAUX SELF-CARE

What I meant when I said "I don't have time" is that every
minute that passes I'm disappointing someone . . .

KATE BAER

Five years ago, burned out at my job and trying to figure out
what I wanted to do next, I decided to spend a week at Esalen
in Big Sur, a gorgeous wellness center set on the cliffs overlook-
ing the Pacific. On my resident's salary this retreat was a splurge,
and I went in taking it *very seriously*. I had certain Big Life Questions I was going to get answered, and I was determined to have
it all figured out by the end of the week. I enjoyed the ocean-side
sulfur baths, the healing massages, and the avocado toast. And
I was militant about journaling and meditating as I searched for
answers to deeper questions that I was convinced this retreat
would provide.

One day, I met a couple in their sixties who had been coming to Esalen every year for decades. Over a lunch of quinoa and butternut squash, they told me that Esalen was their vacation. I noticed myself feeling personally offended and morally outraged— this wasn't a vacation! I was here to do serious work! Looking back, I realize this couple was probably more on track than I was when it comes to what wellness can offer us and what's missing from the equation. Wellness can provide temporary relief, but it can't change us internally unless we do the work of real self-care first.

In this chapter, I'll ask you to take a close look at how faux self-care shows up in your life. Many of us don't recognize the mindset that drives us toward faux self-care. And the first step to change is to bring awareness to what's not working, so in this chapter I'll lead you through the three most common reasons why we turn to faux self-care:

- Escape
- Achievement
- Optimization

It's important to remember that these coping mechanisms are not *bad*—we turn to them for relief during times of stress and overwhelm. By and large, all three of these coping mechanisms come from an understandable desire to control our lives and our circumstances. The issue is they often aren't meeting our deeper needs, and thus end up being Band-Aids instead of sustainable solutions. You might see yourself in more than one of these examples—and that's okay. Typically, we all engage in these activities at different times—myself included. Let's take a look at them together one at a time.

FAUX SELF-CARE AS ESCAPE

My patient Monique, twenty-five, grew up in a tight-knit and controlling religious immigrant family with very high expectations. She also had a disabled father for whom she felt a sense of responsibility. As a nurse, Monique's basic approach to life was to work and work and work and work, until she couldn't take it anymore. Her parents, who had immigrated to the US from the Middle East before Monique was born, modeled this mentality for her as successful small business owners. Every six months Monique would impulsively splurge on a fancy retreat—yoga in Bali, Buddhist Zen meditation in upstate New York, healing with horses in Montana.

In our work together, Monique and I realized that these periodic trips were an escape hatch. Each time she went to a retreat, where she was taken care of by doting staff and where yoga classes and massages were scheduled for her, she not only felt pampered—she felt deeply cared for, albeit by strangers. This was a welcome change for Monique, who in her real life did not allow herself to be cared for by others and instead relished the role of caregiver. Who doesn't love feeling pampered and catered to? But it never translated into real change: Monique would certainly leave her retreats feeling renewed, but she never learned how to integrate any of these routines into her daily life. She would return to her hectic, overscheduled routine and crash.

While aspirational wellness culture sells self-care as an escape from yourself, the truth is that no matter how much faux self-care you do, *you're still you.* Using self-care to escape our regular lives—while temporarily enjoyable—seldom results in lasting change. That's because our true selves are located in our daily choices, and when you use faux self-care as a coping method to escape, you don't have to make any real-world decisions at all.

Consider the typical wellness retreat, like what Monique engaged in periodically or the one I indulged in at Esalen. Beachside yoga at 8:00 a.m., juice bar cleanse at lunchtime, sound healing session before dinner—the agenda is set for you. Depending on your sensibilities (and your budget), it could be a week at a spa or a silent meditation in the mountains or even just a mani-pedi at your local spa. Whatever the setting, you get to "retreat" from the real world and hermit away in a beautiful environment, with healthy food, pleasant surroundings, and a focus solely on self-improvement. Sold as a way to develop a healthier lifestyle and promote wellness-based habits, these temporary escapes allow us to (for a moment, at least) get rid of the tough decisions that need to be made in daily life. And who among us doesn't feel a sense of lightness, even euphoria, when we think about escaping from the daily grind?

This feeling of euphoria—this high—reminds me of something I once overheard a famous rock star speaking about to a group of fans over dinner at—you guessed it—a wellness retreat. He was sober and had been in recovery for years, but he had recently told his therapist he felt like he needed to check into rehab. He wasn't craving drugs or alcohol but rather a week with structures already in place, where he didn't need to make any real decisions. His therapist suggested he go on the wellness retreat.

This makes perfect sense when you consider that wellness retreats are often patterned around 12-step rehab programs, wherein you check into a residential living facility for a few months, get sober, develop healthy new habits and coping skills, and come out into the world with new tools. The bad news is that many people suffering from substance use disorders have trouble staying sober when they are outside the confines of a rehab center. Similarly, many people have trouble continuing to care for themselves properly outside the confines of a wellness retreat.

Whether we know it or not, we turn to this type of faux self-care out of the desire to escape ourselves. Maybe we are running away from grief or destruction due to a failed marriage or the death of a family member. It's understandable—in dark times we are looking for a place of refuge, a bit of rest from life's tragedies. As I mentioned in the introduction, this is why I turned to the cult—I was looking for an escape. Maybe for you it's not a loss that you are running from, but the drudgery of daily life and the fact that every seemingly small decision brings a litany of emotional baggage. "Should I make cupcakes for my kid's school or should I pick some up from the store? If I pick them up from the store, does that mean I'm a bad mom? But I don't have any time to bake cupcakes. Maybe I should skip the workout I had planned for later tonight?" This is internal conflict, and the wellness retreat takes it all away. *Temporarily.*

But the truth is, the trappings of our daily lives, the interpersonal struggles, dealing with the internal conflicts—all of this makes us who we are. It's in the decisions we make in the real world that we mold ourselves and discover what truly matters. I understand that sometimes this just feels way too hard: sorting through the interwoven, complicated threads of what's working in life and what's broken, and then taking action to heal the broken bits, is difficult work. But I assure you that the quick solution never provides sustainable relief.

All of this said, no one should feel ashamed of the urge to escape. As I'll get much more into in the next chapter, women in particular live in a world where we are not given the privilege of time or space for reflection. That's why attendance at wellness retreats is overwhelmingly female.[1] For many of us, the only way to truly hear ourselves think is to get away from everything. And sometimes a retreat or wellness getaway is the very first step in a longer, deeper process of dismantling what's not working in our lives. But a week of self-care in a tropical paradise is unlikely to be a life-reorganizing nirvana that will bring you home shiny and new. The real work begins once the retreat ends.

> ## YOU MIGHT ENGAGE IN FAUX SELF-CARE AS ESCAPE IF YOU IDENTIFY WITH THESE STATEMENTS
>
> - In my daily life, I spend very little time or energy reflecting on my own needs.
> - I'm prone to extreme decisions.
> - I'm an all-or-nothing type of person—either I'm "on," or I'm very, very "off."
> - I feel like a completely different person when I'm on vacation or retreat than in my regular life.
> - I have to get away from everyone else to feel like myself again.

FAUX SELF-CARE AS ACHIEVEMENT

My patient Sharon, forty-five, a white woman who had recently moved to Washington, DC, from New York, built her life around the accumulation of professional successes. She'd been laser focused on her career as a journalist in her twenties and early thirties, rising through the ranks of the newsroom and building an impressive portfolio of assignments. Having come of age in a culture that prizes wellness, she was not someone who ignored her own well-being. Sharon's drive was no doubt influenced by her family of origin—growing up with a single mother who didn't have the opportunity to go to college, Sharon was determined to build a different life for herself than what she experienced as a child. She ate well and was fit, with a membership to Soul-Cycle and a strict diet of clean foods. Twice a year she went to a yoga retreat to recharge. When I met Sharon, though, she had just been laid off, a victim of the volatile media industry.

Without the structure of climbing the professional ladder, she felt lost. So she doubled down and dove headfirst into the world of wellness. She signed up for yoga teacher training, ran a 5K, and read every self-help book she could find. Sharon brought the same laser focus she had utilized in the professional world to her newfound passion for diving deep into "self-care." But despite this frenzy of activity, she still felt isolated and desperate.

Through our work together, we came to understand that the "self-care" Sharon had been engaged in during her time at her job, and even after the layoff, had been a means to an end: Her goal was to win, and to make sure the people in her life knew she was a winner. A selfie followed every yoga class. She obsessively charted her running times on a spreadsheet. Whatever activity she tackled, she had a meticulous internal measuring stick in her mind, and constantly judged herself to see if she measured up. Sharon once revealed to me that after coming home from an exclusive yoga retreat, she didn't feel any better about herself. She had spent the whole week obsessing over holding a headstand and how she looked in her yoga outfits.

That's because Sharon, at her core, had a deep-seated feeling of worthlessness. From a young age she had developed a shield of perfectionism. She had been taught—by her family and the larger culture—that her value was tied to her accomplishments, and no matter how big the win, she was never convinced of her essential, intrinsic worth. Sharon, like many of us, had a hungry ghost inside her, playing tricks on her appetite. In Buddhist philosophy, hungry ghosts are described as skeletal creatures with long, thin necks and large potbellies that are constantly ravenous but never satiated. Here was Sharon, racking up accolades in her work life, running triathlons, and becoming a yoga teacher in the name of "wellness," but never actually feeling a sense of mastery or pride in any of it. That was because her self-care was not grounded in caring or compassion for herself. Instead, the internal voice that drove her to faux self-care was the same internal voice that drove her to stay up late at night working on slide decks: shame.

Sharon is not alone. Many of us grow up with a feeling that we are not good enough just the way we are. But for some women, this deficit is so strong that the need to succeed becomes blinding. A 2016 survey of two thousand women conducted by Weight-Watchers found that women criticized themselves on average eight times a day, with almost half reporting that the self-critical thoughts started before 9:30 in the morning.[2] Sixty percent of women in this survey said they had days in which they criticized themselves nonstop. For women fueled by this kind of self-criticism, as so many of us are, life can feel like a series of races, each of which must be won in order to prove our worth. In this context, faux self-care becomes another activity to excel at, an endeavor to be conquered just like everything else in life. No matter that getting locked into such a cycle is exhausting and does nothing to provide a long-lasting sense of accomplishment or worth.

The drive to succeed, often unconsciously motivated by shame, commonly manifests in a relentless pursuit of faux self-care achievements, none of which actually nourish our true selves. To the contrary, engaging in faux self-care as a coping mechanism in this way only sets us down a path of endless competition, leaving us tired, burned out, and less engaged with what really matters in life.

Unlike women who use faux self-care as an escape, which at least feels like a relief even if it doesn't provide lasting benefits, women who engage in achievement-oriented, performative self-care often buckle under its weight. Take my patient Priya, thirty-two, who was pregnant with her first child when she came to see me. Priya had struggled with an anxiety disorder for most of her adult life. Raised in a South Asian family that prioritized achievement, she had been a straight-A student, went on to a prestigious law school, and joined a top firm in DC before deciding to start a family. Being pregnant added a new layer of expectation to her life, and the way Priya coped with this pressure was to dive into self-care orthodoxy. She obsessively tracked her steps on her Fitbit, religiously monitored her diet, and became zealous about prenatal yoga. She joined several pregnancy-related Facebook groups and took pride in posting pictures and updates on her self-care routine in the groups, even giving advice to other women about how they could practice self-care.

It's not that a healthy diet or physical activity is bad—in fact, they are advisable practices for pregnancy. The lesson here is that Priya was using diet and exercise in the wrong way; the pressure that came with them hurt her and did nothing to improve her emotional well-being. She became panicked when she missed a yoga class and stopped having dinner out with friends to control her diet. She was conflicted about how to balance self-care and the increasing demands of her law firm job. When she developed gestational diabetes in her third trimester, Priya was distraught.

Over many sessions, we uncovered that Priya had been using self-care during her pregnancy as a report card for herself. In her mind, if she was perfect at self-care, it meant she was being a good mom to her baby and thus her delivery would go smoothly and her baby would be safe. Moreover, her self-care performance meant she was mastering motherhood from the beginning, her baby having unconsciously become a reflection of her own desire for success. Through work in therapy, Priya, who had been raised in a chaotic family and endured emotional abuse as a child, came to understand that she was deeply worried that she was going to be a bad mother. The focus on performative self-care as a means of achieving an idealized version of motherhood was the way she defended herself psychologically against her deeper fears.

Like Priya and Sharon, whether it's through a hyperfocus on diet, exercise, or self-improvement, you might be using faux self-care as a measuring stick to track your performance. Our social media–obsessed culture has only intensified this pattern, making sure every faux self-care performance has an audience. Here faux self-care gets wrapped inside the bubble of perfectionism, workaholism, and capitalism. Getting your weekly facial and heading off to your thirty-dollar fitness class is another badge to hold up. Unfortunately, it's impossible for these external activities to sustainably produce the feelings we are looking for them to deliver—worthiness, acceptance, relief. For women who are caught up in this tendency to use faux self-care as a performative defense against inner feelings of unworthiness, the antidote is not more SoulCycle or turmeric lattes. It's the ongoing work of real self-care.

YOU MIGHT ENGAGE IN FAUX SELF-CARE AS ACHIEVEMENT IF YOU IDENTIFY WITH THESE STATEMENTS

- I often have a mental measuring stick running in the back of my mind.
- The thought of losing—in my professional life or personal life—makes me feel sick.
- My self-worth strongly depends on my ability to be seen as a success.
- I often compare myself with others.
- I predictably feel down or worthless when I don't measure up to others.

FAUX SELF-CARE AS OPTIMIZATION

Anita, forty-two, is a Korean American small business owner and a mom of three. Her partner, an airplane pilot, was away for weeks at a time, leaving Anita as the primary household manager. If anyone needed time-saving tools and a focus on organization, it was Anita. When she first came to see me several years ago, she felt disconnected from her life and her kids. She had organized her days to the utmost degree because she felt she had to. If the trains did not run on time, things would most certainly fall apart. Anita therefore approached organizing her household the same way she approached running her small business: with hypercompetence and an emphasis on productivity and control. It wasn't totally surprising; Anita's mother also embodied the role of hyperefficient household manager. For Anita, this meant endless researching and outsourcing, from meal delivery kits and Amazon Dash Buttons to TaskRabbit errand runners. If a "time hack" existed, Anita had tried it in the service of that elusive goal of creating more time for self-care.

You may not think of meal delivery services or other time-saving strategies as faux self-care, and I didn't either at first. But once I came to understand the distinction between *methods* and *principles* from the previous chapter, it was like a light bulb went off in my brain. A meal delivery service is a method, not a principle. What I've come to realize, in working with patients like Anita over the past few years, is that if you look closely, these lifestyle-optimization services, often marketed to busy women who need help in the home, feel uncomfortably similar to the wellness retreat or the fad diet because they are a *method*. They are marketed as *the* solution, as if once you reclaim an extra hour in your day, the hard work is done. And sure, if you have the means, outsourcing can be a helpful way to get by and it can free up much-needed time and space. But in our work together, Anita and I realized that something was off.

You see, even when Anita came up with the "perfect" productivity and organization solution for her family's needs, she didn't feel complete. She still felt like she was *managing* her kids instead of *being with* them. The meal delivery services and time-saving techniques weren't hurting. The problem was that Anita could not turn her brain off and stop herself from thinking about what she could be doing better. When there were items on her list that she didn't get to, she felt uncomfortable and anxious. And even when she did manage to complete all the tasks, she wondered if she was maximizing every possible aspect of her life—for her children, for her partner, and in her career. Was she really being the "best" version of herself? Here, we realized, "best" was synonymous with most efficient, productive, and controlled—not with fulfilled or content.

This kind of focus on efficiency and productivity is a trap that keeps women spinning on a hamster wheel, especially women operating under the weight of the hundreds of weekly tasks required to run a household. It's a fallacy that if we have that one infant sleep gadget or secret to scheduling, then our home and work lives will be transformed. This type of faux self-care optimization is seductive because it whispers to us, "Here's the magic solution." It promises us that someday we can reach a pinnacle of productivity and efficiency such that our life will finally feel like it's fully under our control. But the problem is that we never actually arrive, because we haven't been taught the critical step of identifying the principles.

I'm reminded of former Yahoo CEO Marissa Mayer, who famously said that you could work 130 hours a week if you're efficient about "when you sleep, when you shower, and how often you go to the bathroom." It's the Silicon Valley ethos, the Sheryl Sandberg–espoused "Lean In" culture that says, "Just keep doing more, more, and more, and eventually, you'll get 'there.'" Setting aside the fact that many women aren't afforded the privilege of "leaning in", the problem is that when women buy into the faux self-care complex, they usually don't think deeply about where "there" is. When you use efficiency as a coping mechanism to deal with the chaos of modern life, it's very easy to forget the real point of efficiency: to free up time and space for yourself. *Doing more does not always lead to feeling better.*

Here it can help to understand a bit more about the brain and how it processes emotions. The areas of the brain that you use when you're working on your to-do list are located in the prefrontal cortex. The prefrontal cortex, or the thinking brain, very much wants to make sense of the world—it wants order and control. But the other, more primitive parts of the brain, which include areas like the limbic system, are where we experience connection, empathy, and other important emotions. Interestingly, when I work with women who are burned out, they rarely identify themselves as burned out. Instead, they say, "I need more hours in the day," or "If only I could finish this one big client report, I'll have more time, and things will be okay." Curiously, that's the response from the prefrontal cortex, which just wants to continue getting things done. The feeling parts of the brain, which are screaming from exhaustion, are effectively silenced. Instead of experiencing a healthy range of emotions, women who hyperfocus on productivity ping-pong back and forth between dread and relief.

Admittedly, I struggle with this myself. When I'm looking at a miles-long to-do list, it's like I'm a roadrunner with my sights set on the goal. It's very difficult to tear myself away from that list. While writing this book, for instance, my life partner, Justin, and I were going through in vitro fertilization treatments to start our family. The IVF process is time-consuming and emotionally exhausting. There were moments when I found myself clinging rigidly to the writing schedule I had laid out, desperately wanting to check off chapters and stay on track despite knowing that what I really needed was rest. I realized that I felt more comfortable with productivity because it provided the illusion of control. Letting myself venture off from my to-do list was risky—it meant I had to allow myself to feel, to recognize when my body and mind needed rest, and also to trust that I would be able to recharge and come back to my schedule.

As you might imagine, this inability or unwillingness to access our feelings is a problem. Research suggests that well-being is actually linked to the feeling brain, in particular to feelings of knowing yourself and being seen. In a 2015 study of more than two thousand mothers, Lucia Ciciolla, PhD, a psychologist at Oklahoma State University, found that the well-being of mothers is linked to four factors: feeling unconditionally loved, feeling comforted when distressed, authenticity in relationships, and satisfaction with friendships.[3] Moreover, a 2020 meta-analysis of more than thirty thousand participants found that authenticity, or the degree to which one feels true to oneself, is associated with greater well-being.[4] If you can't access your feelings because you are stuck on the hamster wheel of optimization of faux self-care, it's going to be very difficult to feel loved, comforted, or true to yourself.

The other problem is that if you're like my patient Anita, optimization will often just breed more optimization, as you continue to stay in your prefrontal cortex. In our work together, Anita found that the time she saved through faux self-care time management systems was not used for authentic connection with herself or with others. Instead, it was spent running her prefrontal cortex on overdrive. What Anita really needed—and what so many women need—was to reconnect with her authentic self. She had fallen into the trap of thinking she might become something or someone *else*—someone more productive, someone more shiny. But what if real fulfillment—and real self-care— was about becoming more *herself*?

> ## YOU MIGHT ENGAGE IN FAUX SELF-CARE AS OPTIMIZATION IF YOU IDENTIFY WITH THESE STATEMENTS
>
> - I'm always on the lookout for the next time-saving strategy or solution.
> - I often tell myself that I'll relax once everything else is taken care of.
> - I strongly equate my self-worth with productivity.
> - It's hard for me to spend energy or time on myself when there's a mess in front of me.
> - Problem-solving makes me feel better about myself.

In all three examples in this chapter, my patients were looking for something—a feeling of relief, accomplishment, control—and faux self-care paradoxically ended up taking them *further* from that goal, not closer. This wasn't their fault. My patients (and I) turn to these coping mechanisms because it's what we've been sold, and to be fair, in the short term, all of these methods serve a purpose. However, the issue is that the relief is temporary and external, not long-lasting or internal.

So if faux self-care isn't a sustainable solution, why do we continue to reach for it? For one thing, in a capitalistic society, individual productivity is exalted at all costs, and faux self-care, with its focus on the individual, perpetuates this cycle. Instead of allowing ourselves to be human beings, we are human *doings*—and the self becomes quantified and measured, merely a sum of tasks and accomplishments. But moreover, there is a gender dimension at play as well. The reality is that faux self-care gives us just enough cover to keep us operating in the familiar social and cultural systems that most of us grew up in—the ones where women are the caretakers of other people and their feelings, and in which women are conditioned to prioritize the well-being of others ahead of themselves. It perpetuates the toxic narrative that says making a choice in service of your well-being means you are selfish. Faux self-care as the solution to what ails women exonerates the system of culpability. *But it's not women who are not doing enough—it's the system that is failing us.* Let's take a closer look at this together in the next chapter.

Chapter 3

THE GAME IS RIGGED

YOU'RE NOT THE PROBLEM

Other countries have social safety nets. The US has women.

JESSICA CALARCO

M y patient Mikaleh, forty-one, grew up in a family where she was one of five kids. As the eldest and only daughter, from a young age she was always working around the house and helped to raise some of her siblings. Mikaleh initially came to me for treatment of her anxiety, which she had struggled with for years, though she'd never previously sought professional help. I diagnosed her with obsessive-compulsive disorder and, along with psychotherapy, started her on medication to manage her condition. Over the course of our initial work together, Mikaleh came to understand how important it was for her well-being (and the well-being of her two teenage daughters) for her to have her OCD under control. And, for a period of time, she did well.

Things fell apart, though, when her mother unexpectedly passed away. Mikaleh was devastated, but she had no time to grieve. She went into turbo-powered caregiver mode. Her father, on a fixed income, could not afford to stay in his house, and wanted to move in to Mikaleh's condo. Due to his health issues and financial situation, Mikaleh would need to cover his medical expenses—which were going to be costly and dip into her savings. To swing this, she let go of the community art classes that she had planned to take that semester. She didn't have time for classes anyway, because her dad could do very little for himself. Her mom had been her dad's primary caregiver—three meals a day, laundry washed and folded, the whole nine yards—for more than forty years of marriage. Mikaleh immediately jumped into this role, while also continuing to work full time as a manager for a nonprofit and take care of her two daughters, whom she co-parented with her ex-husband.

All this caregiving for her father was done without much of a second thought, despite the fact that she constantly felt irritated and resentful that not one of her four adult brothers (who all lived close by) offered to help. Burned out and feeling hopeless about what this next phase of her life looked like—one in which she was her father's sole caregiver—Mikaleh was sinking into despair.

Her plight was all too familiar to me. About a year into the COVID-19 pandemic, I'd written an article for *The New York Times*' "The Primal Scream" series—in-depth reporting on how women, in particular mothers employed outside the home, had fared. In this article, I hypothesized that what we had all been calling burnout was actually something different—it was societal betrayal at its most disturbing level. Over the course of the pandemic, the more I heard my patients use the term *burnout*, the more I felt it did not capture the depth of the crisis they were describing. These were women who faced impossible choices: sending their child to school and risking viral exposure or not showing up to work.

This distinction between burnout and betrayal is critical: while burnout places the blame (and thus the responsibility) on the individual and tells women they aren't resilient enough, *betrayal* points directly to the broken structures around them. "This whole pandemic is teaching us all how to roll with the punches," someone wrote to me on social media, "because they are forceful and frequent, and if you don't roll with them, you get steamrolled." When you live inside social structures that make your life harder and force you to make morally impossible decisions, it's not for lack of trying that you feel despair—it's that those systems have betrayed you. In other words, this isn't our fault.

The reality is that these hard knocks were there even before women were pummeled by a global pandemic. I'd seen it with Mikaleh and many others, because the fact of the matter is that the game has long been rigged: our patriarchal society has saddled women with the mental load—the cognitive and emotional burden that comes with running a household—and a series of paradoxical expectations, all of which understandably drive us to embrace faux self-care in our desperate search for a fix.

But it's not us that needs fixing, it's the culture. This chapter not only takes you on a tour of the deeply cruel ways in which our systems are broken but also zooms out for you to see the bigger picture of how a real self-care practice has the potential to enact wider, systemic change. It's my belief that unless a critical majority of women start practicing real self-care, true systems change will not be possible.

While Part II of this book gets into the nuts and bolts of how to put real self-care into action in your own life, through practical tools and exercises, we are taking a pit stop here because I want you to understand what's possible when you practice real self-care. The reason you feel burned out, hopeless, or full of rage is not your fault. And through Mikaleh's story, you'll come to understand that while you are not the problem, you can be part of the larger solution.

A TIPPING POINT

Social and cultural betrayal is no easy entity to tackle in a single chapter or even a single book. Racism, capitalism, colonialism— these are structures that entire graduate programs are constructed around, and I can't do full justice to them here. Luckily, you don't need a PhD to understand that the structures around us aren't working. Most of us see that our systems are not designed for people—they are designed to maximize the objectives of the system itself. So capitalism, for instance, has an objective of making a profit inside the system. White supremacy has the objective of keeping white people in positions of power. Patriarchy runs with the purpose of keeping men at the head of the table. Scholars and thinkers debate which system is the one that creates the most trauma for women, but the purpose of this book is not to be the definitive answer on which system is the worst. Instead, I'm here to show you how our own internal changes, through real self-care, have the power to impact these systems and trigger cascade effects that pay it forward for others.

Mikaleh faced systemic hurdle after hurdle in her life. As a Black woman in America, she learned from a young age that she would need to work three times as hard to garner the respect and success of her non-Black colleagues. This turned out to be true, as Mikaleh spent her college days at a predominantly white institution, where she often faced discrimination and racism. In her current workplace, she frequently worried about how she would be perceived if she spoke up or reflected a differing point of view as one of only two Black women in her office. Our capitalistic society, which values economic gains above all else, made it difficult for Mikaleh to afford childcare after her divorce, when she was raising her girls. Gender inequity and patriarchy had played a role in her life for as long as she could remember, starting out with the large burden of care work that was placed on her shoulders as the only daughter in her family, and now the unspoken expectation that Mikaleh would step in and provide for her father.

Mikaleh is far from the only one of my patients to come up

against systemic obstacles. Every week in my clinical practice I see patients who are butting against one of these cruel social systems, or an intersection of several:

Dana, a Latina physician who found out that a male graduate of her medical school was being offered a higher salary than her, despite them both having the same qualifications and work experience

Julie, a Black woman up for partner at her law firm, who at her review was told by an all-white panel of her peers that people in the firm found her "scary"

Candace, who, having her first child at thirty-nine and single by choice, wondered how she'd handle questions when she inquired about her company's maternity leave policy

Patricia, a woman of color, who was in a battle with her school district about providing one-on-one support for her daughter who has special needs

Smita, who was burned out at her toxic job, but suffered from autoimmune illness as well as depression, and the only way she could afford medical care was to stay in an abusive work environment

Amber, a queer woman who avoided going to a gynecologist for years despite her strong family history of cancer, due to her fear of being traumatized yet again by the medical system

The list goes on and on.

As a psychiatrist, I came to recognize that while my training in medical school and residency gave me the skills to help my patients cope with the anger, grief, and sheer despair that come with contending with structural barriers, I had been taught nothing about the systemic constraints embedded in our society and had to do my own research. Take for example this dramatic statistic that exemplifies so much of what is wrong with our social systems: A study of new parents in Sweden found that when fathers were given thirty days of flexible paid paternity leave benefits, there was a 26 percent decrease in the number of antianxiety prescriptions written for new mothers.[1] In contrast, in America, less than 5 percent of new fathers take more than two weeks of leave.[2] Despite these gaps in social support, structural barriers like those I've described are rarely considered when mental health professionals are working with their patients.

I believe we're at a tipping point as a society—accelerated, no doubt, by the stressors of the pandemic. "We can't wait for help to come and put out the fire, then come to a neat, decade-long consensus about how to rebuild. That point has passed," wrote journalist and author Anne Helen Petersen. "So the question becomes: do we want to continue to prop up the existing system, posting the same articles about our own disintegration? Do our bodies collapse and then our hands live on, just to keep posting these damn articles?"[3] In the past few years, I've noticed a change in my patients, and in my friends and colleagues—and

I have felt it myself. Patients who previously never spoke about issues like racism or income inequality started bringing those social problems up in therapy. Women who are in untenable situations began asking questions about the powers that be. It seems that among women around the world, there is a collective awakening that the jig is up.

This has long been the case for Black and brown women, for LGBTQ folks, for immigrants, and for people living in poverty, and more recently, a wider, more affluent swath of the population has reached this tipping point as well. But with this crisis comes a profound opportunity to do something different—you see, tipping points always come with possibility. Let's look at this together.

BUT WHAT DO I WANT? THE SYSTEMS THAT SILENCE WOMEN

Around the time that things were falling apart, I asked Mikaleh, in the midst of all of these decisions that were seemingly made for her—her dad moving in, taking money out of her savings to pay for his medical bills, spending 24-7 cooking and cleaning and managing his health-care needs—what did *she* want? Not only did she say she had no clue, but she also looked at me like she wanted to punch me (full disclosure: this is not an uncommon feeling for my patients to have).

Mikaleh had been taught from a young age that her worth was in caring for other people, and that her priority should be the needs of others, not herself. In her twenties and thirties, this meant acquiescing to her brothers when they asked to borrow money, and now it meant stepping up and silently bearing the burden of being the sole caregiver for her father. Mikaleh's conditioning led her to feel guilty anytime she voiced her preference and resulted in her feeling selfish for wanting to make herself happy or fulfilled.

This is not unique to Mikaleh: the Bright Horizons 2017 Modern Family Index survey found that in heterosexual couples, working women are two times as likely to be managing the household and three times as likely to be managing kids' schedules as their male partners. In same-sex couples, studies show that once children are in the picture, we also see an unequal division of household labor, with the lower-earning partner bearing a higher burden. In the aftermath of the COVID-19 pandemic, researchers have found that the gender gap in work hours has been exacerbated by 20 to 50 percent,[4] as women were overwhelmingly the ones providing full-time childcare while simultaneously trying to work from home. The United States is the only country among forty-one high-income nations that does not require paid leave for new parents.[5] Mothers are more likely than fathers to say they've been passed over for promotions, and the majority of working parents report that childcare is unaffordable.[6] With the sheer lack of support available, it's no wonder we feel like we're at the end of our ropes.

The lack of care infrastructure impacts all women, as you can see from the examples in this book. But I have noticed that parenthood makes the situation worse, particularly for cis-hetero couples. Inside the family system, this happens for two reasons. First, from day one, the physical and social setup for pregnancy, childbirth, and early parenting is built around a narrative of self-sacrifice (How much pain are you willing to experience to have a "natural birth"? How hard are you working to exclusively breastfeed? Are you going to subject your child to the horrors of sleep training?). Second, even when partners have thoughtful discussions about egalitarian divisions of labor, the most well-meaning expectations fall by the wayside as soon as baby arrives.

The journalist and writer Meg Conley uses the term *multilevel marketing scheme* to describe her experience. "Motherhood in America is a scam," she wrote. "We're told if we work hard enough, raise our children well enough, and faithfully support the American dream, then we'll end up on top. No one ever mentions how the hierarchy of success is shaped like a pyramid."[7] Conley goes on to describe that while motherhood in America doesn't come with a starter kit of supplements to sell or skincare products to bug your Facebook friends about, what it does come with is a dangerously seductive false hope that Conley has seen across multilevel marketing organizations (which, for those who aren't familiar, are very similar to pyramid schemes, wherein only those executives at the top rake in the profits, and the vast majority of consultants, at the bottom of the pyramid, do not see profit, and may go into debt). The people at the minuscule top of the pyramid are largely white and overresourced, whereas the people on the bottom, who make up the majority of the pyramid, are Black and brown, working class or even middle class, and struggling to afford childcare, to send their children to college, or to own a home. The con in this system is the notion that if you keep being a "good mother," taking care of everyone else, someday, somebody will take care of you. It's a system that is set up not for mothers (or people of color or minorities) but instead as a piece of a larger system that continues to hold up the status quo. It's remarkably clear that the people who benefit off of women's labor and self-sacrifice are usually not women.

Mikaleh didn't stop to think about who benefited from the fact that she had cooked for and hosted the family every weekend for the past decade, or the fact that she had planned and executed every birthday and vacation (to the delight of her family, but to the point that she now dreaded holidays). In fact, during her divorce, despite being in dire financial straits herself, Mikaleh lent money to one of her brothers, only to find out that he took his own kids on a trip to Disney with it. Mikaleh was the silent workhorse of the family, yet she didn't reap the benefits of this work—her brothers and her extended family did.

Silvia Federici, PhD, a scholar and theorist of domestic labor, ties women's plight—not just mothers' plight—directly to unpaid domestic labor, which she called *reproductive labor*. Reproductive labor is the work that must be done over and over again, is essential to life, and never has an end point: keeping the pantry stocked, making sure the car has gas, tending to the needs of elderly family members and children. The COVID-19 pandemic brought into broad daylight the distinction of what work is paid and unpaid, and who is doing this labor. Federici writes, "We cannot change our everyday life without changing its immediate institutions and the political and economic system by which they are structured."[8] In other words, the personal is political. Capitalistic systems are built on the model of unpaid reproductive labor; paid work outside the home is exalted. As such, domestic workers are often unpaid, or paid very little, and are disproportionately immigrants and people of color.

The unequal division of reproductive labor extends to the so-called mental load—remembering what's already been done, what needs to be done, and what will need to be done. It's all of the emotional and cognitive energy that goes into managing, planning, coordinating, and anticipating the hundreds of tasks that must take place for a household to run. I often tell my patients that it's like they are the CEOs of their households, as well as the marketing department, the HR rep, and the administrative assistant.

Sociologist and researcher Allison Daminger, PhD, defines the cognitive load (the technical term for the mental load) as "anticipating needs, identifying options for filling them, making decisions, and monitoring progress."[9] Daminger's research found that women do more of the anticipating and monitoring. This aligns with what I see in my clinical practice, wherein my patients lament that while they can delegate to their partners to put out the garbage every week, they have no way of making their partners think ahead about what the kids are going to dress up as for Halloween or when spring-cleaning is happening this year.

Bearing the mental load has very real emotional and psychological consequences for women. A 2019 study published in the journal *Sex Roles* found that bearing a disproportionate amount of the mental load is associated with a strain on well-being and lower relationship satisfaction.[10] It also found that women with higher levels of mental load express greater levels of emotional emptiness; they are more likely to look around at everything they have and think, "Is this all there is?" I see this in my own patients, many of whom twist themselves into knots to scale the professional ladder and keep up with the unrelenting demands of motherhood, only to feel like they're not doing anything quite right and resentful that this is their burden to bear.

Mikaleh was the poster child for a larger-than-life mental load, as she navigated tending to her father's medical needs, keeping her two teenagers doing well in school, and managing her responsibilities at work. Her mind was a blur of questions like, "Does Dad have any refills left on his prescriptions or do we need to call his doctor? When does the school math specialist need that paperwork so we can start tutoring? Is the water heater on the fritz again?" and so on. To be fair, it's also Mikaleh who gets blamed for domestic mishaps, not her kids' dad, so it's no wonder she's the one doing the worrying.

Gloria Steinem famously wrote: "Power can be taken, but not

given. The process of the taking is empowerment in itself."[11] The hard truth is that if any of this—the marketing scheme, the unequal division of reproductive labor, the overwhelming mental load—is to be fixed, it's on women to do it. You might be thinking, "Jeez it's really not fair, we have enough to deal with already!" You're right—it's not fair. *And* the reality is that people who are in power rarely give up that power. The class of people who benefit from the systems as they currently exist are not going to wake up one morning and decide they want a more equitable system. The people at the top *do* respond to pressure from the bottom, yet the people at the bottom don't have time or mental energy to fight back or to change how they interact or question why things are done the way they are done. This is how oppressive systems work and the reason they stay functioning. Thus, we need people from the bottom (women, people of color, queer and minoritized people) to rise up and, when they reach those levels of power, to start making changes. And that is precisely what real self-care is about.

THE PARADOX OF CHOICE

At this point, some might be tempted to argue that if women spent less time worrying about putting their kids in matching outfits or making sure the house was Pinterest-level decorated, maybe they would have time for real self-care. In other words, are women choosing this reality? As per usual, it's a bit more complicated than yes or no.

Martha Beck, PhD, is a sociologist, life coach, and author who has spent the past thirty years studying how culture impacts women.[12] In her book *The Way of Integrity*, she argues that what defines a culture is a shared set of values—for example, in our culture we value when people wait in line for their turn, or when they use utensils to eat spaghetti. There are bigger values as well—work hard, pull yourself up by your bootstraps, but wait, also be a team player, and also wait, you're solely responsible for your own destiny. Notice the contradictions? As we see time and time again, women are pulled in two opposing directions—asked to be selfless and accommodating to the needs of others and, simultaneously, to excel professionally and personally.

It's also important to consider that it's not as simple as making the "right" choices; instead, we must reflect critically on what choices are *even available* to us. Mikaleh, for example, had to choose between going back to school and chipping in for her father's medical bills. She was forced to choose between competing values: on the one hand, she wanted to be a selfless daughter who provided for her father, but on the other hand, she valued lifelong learning. Deep down, Mikaleh knew this creative outlet for herself was important to her own well-being and her mental health. When she signed up for the art classes, she found herself feeling enthusiastic in a way that she had not for years. Yes, technically she had a choice. But that choice was between duty and her own well-being.

A friend recently shared a similar story that you can probably relate to—though with the stakes not quite as high as Mikaleh's.

Her family was invited to a potluck holiday party. She signed up to bring dessert and on the day of the party had to cut her workday short to bake a cake. This meant her husband had to step in and pick up their kids. The morning of, he remarked to my friend, "You're making our life more difficult—we could have just taken a store-bought cake." In that moment, my friend felt that she couldn't win: She knew the hostess had put care and effort into this party, and a store-bought cake would stick out like a sore thumb. Nobody would blame her husband if the cake was purchased, not homemade—they would look to her failing as a woman. And it was true that it made their Friday afternoon more complicated. No matter what, somehow, it was still all her fault.

"Modern women's dilemma is a koan," Dr. Beck told me, invoking the Buddhist concept of a riddle that defies logic. "It's an unsolvable problem."[13] She believes women are playing a game they cannot win. We are our society's scapegoats, asked to complete the impossible task of squaring the contradictions of our entire culture.

The more you give to your job, the more guilt you feel at home. The more you excel at home, the more behind you feel at work. Women are squeezed into a smaller and smaller corner, until there is no room to feel much of anything aside from anger or helplessness. Faux self-care is an illusion sold to women to, as Beck calls it, "reconcile the irreconcilable." As women, when we experience this conflict, our instinct is to blame ourselves and assume we should be able to figure out the "right" answer. But, alas, it doesn't work because the rules are contradictory—there is no *right* answer! Instead, we internalize the paradox as guilt, self-doubt, even despair.

The research backs this up. A Mercer University study of thirty-one moms explored self-care practices in the postpartum period.[14] The study found that women expressed two contradictory themes that pulled them in opposite directions: Self-care is of primary importance *and* selflessness is synonymous with motherhood. On the one hand, self-care is seen as a woman's responsibility and part of living up to society's expectations of taking care of our individual needs. On the other hand, selflessness, especially in the service of children or partners, is viewed as the feminine ideal. It's these contradictory cultural values, in which women are expected to be both self-sacrificing as well as professionally ambitious, that faux self-care completely bypasses. You can't self-care yourself out of a forty-hour workweek with no childcare. Buying a new day planner and going to yoga won't change the fact that you bear a disproportionate share of the mental load.

It feels like a catch-22, right? If we get stuck in a feeling of powerlessness about how the system is stacked against us, change does not occur. If we throw ourselves into faux self-care and align ourselves with the capitalistic and patriarchal structures that be, we internalize the sickness and exonerate the system.

We can't do either of these things.

Instead, for true change to happen—for real self-care to lead all of us to a more equitable and equal social structure—we as women must do two things:

- embrace internal change
- cultivate what's called dialectical thinking

On the first, Einstein said, "a new type of thinking is essential if mankind is to survive and move toward higher levels." The dizzying values, contradictions, and impossible expectations put on women, quite simply, make no sense at all. We cannot look to outside structures or rules to save us because the logic[15] on the outside is deeply flawed. So, we must aim for something completely different—a solution that challenges everything we have come to know. *Real self-care is an internal solution: it's about changing your internal reality—or your consciousness.*

So, before Mikaleh could take action, she first had to give herself the permission to make an internal change. Through our work together, Mikaleh came to understand that she valued her mental health as one of her top priorities. She showed up as a better mother when she was taking care of her mental health. She was on top of her game at work when her OCD was treated. Mikaleh did not want to go back to a life where her anxiety was in control. She comprehended for the first time that nobody else was going to give her permission to take care of herself; it would have to be something she decided, even if it meant letting others down. This was not simply squeezing in a yoga class; instead, Mikaleh began to think differently about her health and how much space *she* occupied in her life.

From here, Mikaleh began to cultivate dialectical thinking, which means acknowledging that two opposites can be true at the same time. There is even a specific type of therapy called DBT, or dialectical behavior therapy, that teaches this skill.[16] The founder of DBT, Marsha Linehan, refers to it as an integration of opposites. Mikaleh was faced with a dialectic: she loved her father dearly *and* realized that she alone could not care for him. Reconciling this dialectic for Mikaleh meant that *both* of these statements were true. She did not have to choose—she could live with both of these truths holding equal weight in her life. This was tough for Mikaleh because growing up, love was equated with self-sacrifice. Once she came to understand that she could live her life with both truths occupying space in her mind, she felt lighter. She felt empowered to engage with herself and with her family with less fear, and finally began allowing her own needs and preferences to play a larger role in her decisions.

THE REVOLUTIONARY POSSIBILITY OF REAL SELF-CARE

Mikaleh came to understand that she had reached a tipping point of her own. Managing her father's doctor appointments and his complicated regimen of medications, and pinching pennies to pay his bills (on top of all of her other responsibilities) triggered Mikaleh's OCD in full force. She tried to treat it without taking time off, but she found herself showing up late for work, calling in sick, and turning in reports late; something had to give. If she did nothing, she'd likely end up demoted or fired from her job. If she took a risk and applied for a leave of absence, she might miss out on the promotion she was due for the following year, or worse, be pushed out of her job.

Ultimately, Mikaleh was able to see this tipping point as an opportunity to make a different and new type of decision for herself. She took a risk and requested a monthlong leave of absence from work to manage her mental health. It was grueling navigating the red tape of applying for short-term disability. But she was fortunate that her workplace had a helpful HR department.

Several curious things happened after Mikaleh took this mental health leave. First, having the month to see me consistently helped get her OCD under control. It also gave her the space to reflect on her relationships with her brothers and work up the strength to ask them to pitch in financially to care for her father. It further gave her time to navigate the maze of her father's insurance benefits and find that they had coverage for five hours a week of home health support, which was a small but powerful relief for her.

Mikaleh made the choice to tell a couple of close friends at work that she had been struggling with mental health issues and that's what led to her taking time off. She connected with a team member whose son had OCD that was long undiagnosed, and they put together a presentation about the symptoms of OCD. Then, together, they approached the leadership of the organization to see if they could streamline the process of taking a mental health leave. Six months later, they had started a group within the organization for people suffering from mental health conditions or supporting family members with mental health concerns. Mikaleh soon found that junior members of the organization were reaching out to her for resources when they were struggling. She advocated for this new role she had taken on within her company to be a line item in her pay structure. The next year when she was up for a promotion, the leadership remarked that her time off was not evidence of failure; it was actually aligned with her strengths and shifted the company's culture.

You may think, "Well I don't have an employer nearly as understanding as Mikaleh's." Or maybe you're thinking, "My family would never chip in financially to help out in a crisis." In other words, you might be thinking, "This system completely sucks. Why don't we just BURN IT ALL DOWN?" Believe me—I get that. And for better or worse, I've been there and I'm here to tell you: burning it all down never works in the long run. Remember, I burned my life down and joined a group dedicated to female orgasm, so I can attest from personal experience that it doesn't work. Burning it all down—whether it's your life or the system— doesn't fix the problem. It's just another way of running from your problems, only to find them staring back at you in the mirror. To truly change the system, we must work from the inside out, starting right where we are—in our current lives.

Real self-care is still work. But, as you'll see, it's less about adding something to your list and more about seeing your place in the world, your family, and your relationships differently. And when you engage in self-care this way, you are living a small revolution and remaking the system. Again, take to heart the words of Audre Lorde: "Caring for myself is not self-indulgence, it is self-preservation, and that is an act of political warfare."[17] We have reached a tipping point, wherein the old ways of being and working are clearly not the path forward. The time has long since come for us to take back our power. And in fomenting a small revolution inside yourself, you'll be contributing to the wider, systemic revolution.

WHAT ABOUT MEN?

A friend recently told me a story about how she sent her husband to the dentist with her kids for their regular cleaning, and the dentist chastised him with, "Mom should be here for this." Whenever I write or speak about systems issues, the first comment I get is about men. It goes something along the lines of "Yeah but if men just pulled their weight, then women inside these relationships wouldn't feel like such crap."

Alas, the answer to this question (like the answer to most questions) is complicated. I spoke to writer and journalist Brigid Schulte, director of the Better Life Lab at New America, whom I met through our work as part of the CareForce, a multidisciplinary coalition of researchers, scholars, business leaders, and change makers advocating for gender justice and caregiver policy change. Brigid studies gender and care work, and in particular, her organization has researched how to bring men into household work. New America surveyed nearly three thousand adults in 2019 and found that more than 80 percent of women reported that they believe men and women should equally share household work, but only 46 percent of those surveyed said care work was shared evenly.[18] While it's easy to become enraged at men and to point fingers, the reality is that the problems are much bigger than a battle between genders. Brigid points out that raging at men is a distraction. She says, "they are just as stuck as women and it's the system that we should all be enraged by." Instead of being pitted against each other, we need people from all points on the gender spectrum to challenge our existing social systems if we want to see change.[19]

Brigid's take reflects what I see in my practice as well. There are many men in cisgender heterosexual relationships who are pulling their weight in terms of household responsibilities and child-rearing, only for an incident like what happened to my friend at the dentist to occur. Groups like the CareForce are fighting to bring care work into mainstream policy conversations. Brigid suggests that there are three levers we can pull—public policy, workplace policy, and implementing systems inside the family. For example, in the workplace, companies can incentivize all workers, regardless of gender, to take paid family leave, or enact policies that promote standard flexible work by default so that those with disabilities or caregiving responsibilities are not singled out. I view real self-care as one of these systems wherein, as you'll learn in the rest of the book, you are implementing a process for yourself that then has a cascading effect for others in your life.

THE PATH FORWARD

What if instead of berating ourselves for not being enough, we recognized that it's the systems that have failed us?

What if we stopped reaching for the quick-fix solutions and did the internal work that stays with us forever, that is truly our own, in a way that a product can never be?

What if we thought about self-care as an internal, quiet process that has the power to create an external and dramatic change?

If these statements resonate with you and if you're ready to take the risk and dive into a whole new paradigm of real self-care, keep reading to find out exactly how to make this happen.

PART II

REAL SELF-CARE
IS AN INSIDE JOB

Chapter 4

TAKING BACK THE REINS

THE FOUR PRINCIPLES
OF REAL SELF-CARE

Anyone who is interested in making change in the world
has to learn to take care of herself, himself, theirself.

ANGELA DAVIS

I f real self-care isn't a life hack, a wellness retreat, or the latest
fad, then what is it? Again, real self-care is not a noun, it's a
verb—an ongoing internal process that guides us toward profound emotional wellness and reimagines how we interact with
others. It requires self-knowledge, self-compassion, and ultimately, the willingness to make difficult decisions. What I've
come to learn through working with my patients, reading the
scientific research on well-being, and reflecting on my personal
therapeutic journey is that the twenty-first-century definition of
real self-care corresponds most closely to a concept called *eudaimonic well-being.*

EUDAIMONIC WELL-BEING: DOING WHAT MATTERS MOST

Most of us are striving for a life in which we can do what matters most to us, and in which we feel we have real choices about how we spend our time and energy. But we get bogged down in that pursuit—confused about where exactly we're headed.

Research on well-being is divided into two distinct theories of how to go about living a good life: the hedonic approach and the eudaimonic approach. Hedonic well-being focuses on the feeling states of happiness and pleasure—like Monique's wellness retreats. In many respects, faux self-care—the diets, the cleanses, the retreats, the life hacks—is aligned with this hedonic approach, with its focus on what feels good in the moment and on escaping life's difficult situations. Don't get me wrong— we all need escape every once in a while, and the ability to afford such hedonism is a privilege.

Eudaimonic well-being, in contrast, focuses on deriving meaning and having our actions be congruent with our values; it is the feeling that our lives are imbued with purpose.[1] Instead of prioritizing pleasure or happiness, eudaimonic well-being emphasizes personal growth, acceptance of your authentic self, and connection to meaning. Not surprisingly, it is linked to better health outcomes, including improved sleep,[2] longer life span,[3] and lower levels of inflammation.[4] All the good stuff we're looking for, right?

Cultivating eudaimonic well-being isn't straightforward, however. It looks different for everyone because the decisions we make to achieve it are dependent on our personal beliefs and values. For some people, it might mean letting go of demanding fitness goals and spending weekends volunteering for a worthwhile cause. For others, it might mean investing time and energy into feeling more connected with their children. For still others it might mean switching to a career more aligned with their values. But what is similar across individuals is that each person is doing what matters to them and understands the meaning behind how they spend their time. Far more than any passing fad or wellness retreat, this is real self-care.

The million-dollar question, of course, is how do we distinguish real self-care—the practices that lead us to eudaimonic well-being—from the coping mechanisms of faux self-care discussed in Part I? How do we ensure that we are practicing the kind of real self-care that is likely to lead to profound fulfillment? The answer is to take the time to align our self-care practices with the following four principles, all based in moving toward eudaimonic well-being.

Let's take a look at each of the principles of real self-care, one by one.

Real Self-Care Requires Boundaries and Moving Past Guilt

At its core, real self-care is ultimately about decision-making. In order to make decisions that foster eudaimonic well-being, you must be assertive in prioritizing your own needs and desires. To do that, you must learn to say no and to set boundaries. This often means balancing the needs of people close to you, like your partner's preference or your children's needs, with your own desires and needs. In this process, you must learn to stop being controlled by feelings of guilt, which are inevitable but can be managed.

Real Self-Care Means Treating Yourself with Compassion

Once you've gotten a grasp on how to set boundaries, the next step of real self-care is to insert compassion into how you speak to yourself. Practicing real self-care means looking honestly and unflinchingly at what you need (and what you want) and giving yourself permission to have it. This is only possible if you cultivate compassion for yourself. Included in practicing self-compassion is the work of overcoming common patterns like Martyr Mode and looking closely at how you talk to yourself.

Real Self-Care Brings You Closer to Yourself

While faux self-care takes you further from yourself, real self-care always brings you closer to the most authentic version of yourself. It's a process of getting to know yourself—your *real* self—including your core values, beliefs, and desires. It's an internal decision-making process that requires introspection, honesty, and perseverance. You'll know you're practicing real self-care when it feels like your outsides are matching your insides.

Real Self-Care Is an Assertion of Power

While faux self-care only serves to keep women small, real self-care is about making yourself bigger, and in turn, shifting long-standing systems of power. While women have long been taught to wait for permission to exert this type of control over our lives, we are the only ones who can give ourselves permission to practice real self-care. Make no mistake: Real self-care, wherein you look inside yourself and make decisions from a place of reflection and consideration, is an assertion of power. It means facing, straight on, the toxicity and trauma that our culture brings to women. It's about saying this is what works for me, and this is what doesn't. It's having the audacity to say, "I exist and I matter." These are revolutionary acts—and it's only when a critical mass of women do this internal work that we will come to collective change in our world.

These four principles overlap, and each step relies on the learnings of the principle that came before it—as you'll see through my patient Clara's story.

When Clara, forty-five, came to see me, she had been working as a public school teacher for a decade. Clara came from a long line of educators—her father had been a professor in their home country of Colombia and her mother worked at a daycare center. Yet after years of budget cuts and setbacks at her public school, Clara felt burned out and drained. There were still moments of joy to be had, like when a student made progress or a family sent her a heartfelt thank you note. But inside, Clara knew she could not go another decade pouring all of herself into her work with nothing left over for herself. She had tried a wide range of faux self-care practices and undergone resiliency training, but nothing had helped for any sustainable period of time. So we began our work identifying how Clara could take better care of herself while working in this profession that she so clearly loved.

Over several months of therapy, which involved looking carefully at which parts of her job brought her joy and which brought her frustration, we identified that one of Clara's core values is agency—feeling it in herself and supporting it in others. When school administrators took away her agency by second-guessing her decisions—something that had been happening more and more often—she felt demoralized and small. But when she helped her students gain confidence in their abilities—when she nourished their agency—she felt like she was living in alignment with her purpose.

Clara eventually made a plan to leave the school and start her own business providing tutoring to students with learning disabilities. This involved overcoming feelings of guilt (over wanting to leave the public school environment) and envy (of teachers who had been brave enough to leave the system and take control of their own lives). But by identifying her values and reflecting on the feelings underneath, Clara was able to make the leap and start her own business.

Now, this doesn't sound like the self-care so many of us are used to—there is no product to buy or wellness practice to credit. Real self-care is not a *thing* to do, it's a *way* to be. If you break it down, you'll see that Clara's decision-making process not only promoted eudaimonic well-being but was in perfect alignment with the principles of real self-care: It required setting boundaries (she would not continue to be treated poorly by the administration). It involved treating herself with compassion (she had to accept her feelings of guilt and envy). It brought her closer to herself (she gained a newfound understanding of the importance of agency in her life). And it involved an assertion of power (she had to both quit her job and start a new business).

Each of the chapters in Part II will explore one of the four principles in depth, providing concrete advice and exercises for putting the principle into action as you begin to develop your real self-care practice.

WAIT, MORE WORK?

If you're anything like the women in my practice, as you read through the Four Principles of Real Self-Care and Clara's story, you might be thinking, "Ugh, more work! Didn't we just spend the first part of the book talking about how women are doing too much already, and aren't even being paid for it?"

Yes, dear reader, you're right. I am asking you to do more

work—you caught me. And before you throw this book across the room, let me explain. The tools I will teach you in the rest of the book are based on a type of behavioral therapy called ACT, which stands for acceptance and commitment therapy.[5] ACT is different from other types of therapy because it starts with the assumption that we all suffer in life, and that there is no way around said suffering. Instead of focusing on getting rid of bad thoughts or difficult feelings, ACT teaches us to move forward *despite* the suffering, by taking action toward what matters most to us in life. ACT is a type of therapy that supports living a more eudaimonic life—one in which your insides match your outsides, and how you spend your time and energy aligns with your values. This requires emotional and mental labor on your part—you'll have to ask yourself tough questions and be willing to have hard conversations with people you care about. I can't pretend that it's easy but, trust me, it *does* work.

There might be some of you who are still tempted to throw up your hands at all of this. I don't blame you and I'm not stopping you. I encourage you to take all the time you need. Watch ten seasons of *The Great British Bake Off* if that's what you're craving, jump into a saltwater immersion tank, try Keto. Once you've had your fill of the wellness solutions, see how you feel. Ask yourself how it's worked for you. Most of us end up at this place, reading a book like this (or, let's be honest, *writing* a book like this), because we have tried everything and it hasn't worked. You're very likely here because you are open—maybe even desperate—to try something new. Most people come to this work once they've exhausted all the faux self-care options and have nothing left to lose. Like the practice of real self-care itself, choice is of paramount importance. You don't need to work through all of the principles in one day. Take breaks when it gets too hard and come back when you can. This is a gentle approach, not one that asks for striving or self-flagellation.

HOW TO PRACTICE REAL SELF-CARE WHEN YOU SUFFER FROM A CLINICAL MENTAL HEALTH CONDITION

Wellness has gotten things a bit mixed up when it comes to mental health and self-care. Right now there's a misconception that you can self-care yourself out of major depressive disorder or post-traumatic stress disorder. However, mental health conditions are neurobiologic and require trained professionals to provide psychotherapy and, sometimes, psychotropic medications to help you feel better. Instead of thinking of self-care as a tool to treat a specific condition, think of it more like a spot test, to see how you are doing. If you know that your daily walk in the dog park with Fido is your nourishing time, yet you find that you just can't bring yourself to take the dog out or if your guilt is so intrusive and constant you feel completely powerless to stop it, that could be a sign that you need to seek professional help. Once your psychiatric condition is treated, then it becomes possible to enact the principles of real self-care, and to put practices in place. I've lived this personally—I've struggled with clinical anxiety and depression in the past and had to seek treatment for those conditions before I could begin the self-guided work of real self-care.

The Three Yellow Flags on Your Real Self-Care Path

As you go through the principles of real self-care, it's important to be clear as to what real self-care is not. There are three yellow flags, and it's tempting to get caught up in them, fall away from the path of real self-care, and go right back to faux self-care. Pressure to revert to a cookie-cutter, one-size-fits-all mentality comes at us from all sides, so it's worth stopping here to put the three flags on your radar.

Real Self-Care Is Not without Risk

To practice real self-care, you must be willing to make yourself vulnerable—whether that means having uncomfortable conversations to set boundaries or making the clear and deliberate choice to prioritize one aspect of your life over another. The good news is that these leaps of faith pay off in the long run: every decision that you make in the service of real self-care takes you further away from the oppressive systems that keep you down and brings you closer to who you are. There is always a cost—whether it's financial, social, or emotional—*and* there is also a gain, in the form of emotional well-being, ownership of your time and energy, and ultimately, shifts in your relationships.

So, it makes sense that in order to do this work, we must cultivate courage. In her TED Talk called "The Power of Vulnerability,"[6] which has been viewed more than fifty million times, Brené Brown, PhD, makes the connection between risk and courage. Brown has spent the past two decades studying courage, vulnerability, shame, empathy, and what separates people who take risks from those who do not. Ultimately, Brown found that "these folks had, very simply, the courage to be imperfect.... They were willing to let go of who they thought they should be in order to be who they were."

Building a life in which you take care of yourself will always come with risks—anyone who tells you that you can have it without a cost has an agenda to sell you. The good news is that the benefits come not only to you, as we saw with Clara, but also to those around you, and even the systems that you work inside. And the fact that our systems are so stacked against us is precisely why we must have the courage to face the inner work of real self-care.

Real Self-Care Is Not a Religion

Especially in times of social chaos or turmoil, it's natural to look toward gurus or external sources of authority for the Answer. I'm perhaps most passionate about this yellow flag due to my personal history. Anyone who tells you that there is *only* one path to well-being should trigger the tiny hairs on the back of your neck. Real self-care requires us to subvert the paradigm that there is one answer to wellness. As you move through the tools in this book, remember that what I'm offering here is not canon. You will question my assertions, you will find that some of it is not for you, and you will not follow it to a tee. That means you are doing it right. You are not meant to use this book as a bible, because the entire premise of real self-care is that we as human beings can never expect to find a one-size-fits-all solution. We have to be careful not to become fanatical about any particular practice. We're all vulnerable to the seduction of so-called gurus, but it's especially true the more our social structures fail us.

Real Self-Care Is Not a Destination

When I found a publisher for *Real Self-Care* in 2021, I said to my therapist, Christie, how am I going to write this book? Am I qualified to take this on? I'm a self-described workaholic. Self-care is one of the most difficult propositions for me. I ended up falling for Big Wellness in the worst way—I joined a cult! With compassion, Christie, who has been by my side since my early days of leaving the cult, said, "Pooja, I have a feeling that writing this book is going to be a process of self-discovery and healing for you." She was right.

Yes, I'm a psychiatrist, so I have the clinical training and the expertise, but as many of you know, taking your own advice is much more difficult than doling it out. I'm not here to give you advice from the top of the mountain. I'm here as a fellow traveler alongside you. And certainly there are days, weeks, even months when I fall back into my masochistic ways, beat myself up, forget to say no, and lose sight of what's most important. I have guides who help me get back on track—like Christie, my family, friends, and colleagues who support me. I lean on this team, and I pick myself back up and try again. That's the work of real self-care. There is no perfection, and there is also no checking it off the list and calling it done.

If it's disheartening to you to learn that real self-care is not a neat and tidy solution, take some solace—remember back in Chapter 1 we talked about how faux self-care prescribes methods, whereas real self-care focuses on principles? This is critical because living by your principles is a lifelong process. Your circumstances will constantly change—whether you're having a baby, transitioning into a new job, or navigating the challenges of caring for aging family members. You will constantly need to learn how to apply the principles of real self-care to novel situations, but you will become more practiced and confident in applying these principles. A tidy solution could never work for the long haul, and folks, we are in it together for the long haul.

CELEBRATE REAL SELF-CARE FAILS

Using these principles—even imperfectly—to guide your actions moves you in the direction of real self-care. There is no pressure to "get it right" and do it perfectly all the time. There will be situations in which you look back and say to yourself: "Wow, I really should have said no to that giant time suck of a work project," or "Jeez,

I spent an hour berating myself because I forgot to sign my kid up for summer camp." This is normal and okay and expected. Not only that, it doesn't take away from your progress of real self-care. This is the beauty of an internal, self-guided framework—it's nonbinary, and simply by keeping these principles as a guide in the back of your mind, you're doing enough.

Chapter 5

REAL SELF-CARE
REQUIRES BOUNDARIES

MOVING PAST GUILT

To free us from the expectations of others, to give us back to ourselves—there lies the great, the singular power of self-respect.

JOAN DIDION

M y patient Angela, thirty-two, had a tendency to be the fixer in her household. Run out of toilet paper? She'd jump up for the Target run. Boyfriend locked out of the apartment? She'd hop in a cab to save him. One day she shared a pretty revealing story with me. Angela and her boyfriend had recently moved in together and decided to adopt a puppy. She was juggling working part time as an executive assistant and getting her master's degree in social work, and she was approaching her finals week. Not only that, on weekends, she had to do the clinical rotations required to finish her degree.

One Saturday, her boyfriend was out with friends while she

was at her clinical site. That morning they'd made a plan for him to be home by 3:00 p.m. to take the puppy, Elie, for a walk. She received a text from him at 2:45 p.m. saying that his buddy wanted to grab dinner together, so he wouldn't be able to make it home to walk Elie. He wanted to know if Angela could finish up her work early and make it home. Angela immediately rushed to the rescue, quickly finishing the last of her charting and asking her supervisor if she could make up her evening clinical shift the following weekend.

In our session that week, Angela shared this anecdote as an example of how, while her partner had dropped the ball, she was able to save the day. She was feeling good about her ability to juggle more than seemed humanly possible. She explained, "I know I'll have to make up that evening shift, but we don't have plans next weekend, so it worked out."

I asked Angela why she decided to say yes to her boyfriend's request when they had already made a plan that he would be responsible for Elie that afternoon. Didn't this change in plans make more work for her? Angela was a little taken aback.

"Well, my supervisor was really flexible and so it's fine."

"But didn't you come up with a plan that morning, and hadn't he agreed to be responsible for Elie that afternoon?"

Angela, looking sheepish, said, "I guess it didn't occur to me to say no to him. . . ."

I pushed her a little further. "I'm noticing that we have spent so much of our time together talking about how important your master's program is to you. What do you think of the fact that you were willing to quickly drop your priority so your boyfriend could spend more time with his friend?"

In my practice, I see many women like Angela who struggle to set limits with their partners, families, and even friends. While Angela's situation may seem extreme, you might notice varying degrees of this behavior in your own life. For instance, like Angela, in the heat of the moment you might not recognize setting a boundary is an option. Or perhaps you're aware that you want to say no but are uncomfortable setting a boundary that might lead to conflict. Or perhaps you feel too much guilt to firmly communicate your choice. Failure to set boundaries not only mires Angela and women like her in unfulfilling activities, it also prevents them from having the mental and emotional bandwidth to engage in real self-care practices.

The first principle of real self-care, then, is setting boundaries. Boundaries are the cornerstone; without them, none of the rest of the work can happen. Real self-care is all about making space for *you*—your thoughts, feelings, and priorities in life. Most of my patients need to fight their way to having this space, because they don't see their time and energy as belonging to them. And, again, this isn't their fault. Our entire system is built on the premise that women's time—and especially the time of Black and brown women—doesn't belong to them. Setting boundaries is how we take our time, energy, and attention back.

WHAT EXACTLY ARE BOUNDARIES?

Think of boundaries as the energetic space between two people. Lest that sound a little too woo-woo, let me explain. When I was a new faculty member at George Washington University's Department of Psychiatry and Behavioral Sciences, my mentor, Dr. Lisa Catapano, took me out for lunch. She had grown to be a friend as well as a mentor over the years, and we'd had many conversations about how to navigate the tricky terrain of being a woman in a male-dominated profession like medicine. Dr. Catapano, in her confident and tell-it-like-it-is manner that I've always found reassuring and compassionate, gave me a piece of advice that dramatically shifted my views about professional boundaries: *You don't have to answer your phone.*

I was a bit stunned. This was the exact opposite of the training I'd received as a medical student and a resident. In those days, the dogma was "Be available at all times, answer your pages immediately." That mentality of always being "on" carried over even when I wasn't on call at the hospital.

"Let it go to voicemail," Dr. Catapano said of my office line, "and listen to the message. See what the person wants and then take a couple of minutes to decide what you want to do."

The idea that I not only was allowed to take time, but that in that space I could decide the best response, was nothing short of revolutionary to me. It didn't matter whether the caller was the front desk staff telling me they had paperwork they needed me to sign or a patient who needed to reschedule an appointment. When I picked up my phone, I felt pressured to say yes and react. Not answering my phone and letting it go to voicemail gave me time and space to craft my response and be strategic about my time and energy.

My boundary was in the *pause*.

Inside the pause, it was up to me to decide how to answer. I could say, "Sure, let me take care of that right away." Or I could say, "I'm back-to-back with patients all day. Can you put it in my mailbox and I'll look at it tomorrow?" As a doctor, there are times when patients need me urgently. But by taking the step to let my phone go to voicemail, I'm not abandoning or ignoring anyone—I'm giving myself the time to respond instead of reacting. In fact, by taking ownership of my attention, I actually *improve* my ability to be available for my patients in those rare cases of emergency.

Setting boundaries is about recognizing you have a choice and communicating it. But before you can get to either of those things, you need to grapple with a gigantic obstacle that almost always rears its head: other people's feelings. Because when you communicate a boundary, something tricky happens. Whether the boundary is set with a friend, a family member, or an elementary school's PTA, there will likely be consequences, real or imagined. For instance, there are some who would recoil at my decision not to answer my office line. But boundaries are not cocreated. Other people will have their own feelings about your boundaries, but they cannot create them. A boundary is about what *you* need to interact in the world.

The tension between what you need and what other people in your life expect of you is at the core of why setting boundaries is difficult for many women, and so let me make the link plainly: *Boundaries are hard not because you can't identify yours, but because you are worried about the backlash.* Remember this language and come back to it when coaching yourself through the difficult work of setting boundaries.

In this next section, I will share an exercise you can use to assess your real self-care level. Then, after you are equipped with this knowledge, the rest of the chapter will guide you through my framework for setting boundaries, which contains specific techniques for dealing with guilt, letting go of what other people think, and making requests. At the end of the chapter, I'll answer common questions about setting boundaries that I often see in my practice.

THE REAL SELF-CARE THERMOMETER

When I assess a patient's ability to practice real self-care, I don't worry about whether they go to yoga every week or whether they are drinking enough water every day. Instead, over the years, I've found that my patients' capacity to recognize that they have choices and their ability to communicate those choices is a fairly reliable measure of how well they take care of themselves. So, to start our work, I've created an exercise called the Real Self-Care

Thermometer. The Real Self-Care Thermometer will help you measure your capacity to identify and communicate your boundaries in a number of commonly thorny life circumstances. Score yourself at the end to see which category you fall into (Red, Yellow, or Green). While each question in the Real Self-Care Thermometer may not exactly match your life circumstances, use your best guess as to how you might respond if it did.

Question 1

You're on a weekend getaway with your closest friends. It took a year to organize everyone's schedules and you've been looking forward to it for months. You're just about to step into a yoga class when you get a text from your boss, who knows you're offline for the weekend, asking if you could be so kind as to forward the spreadsheet you've been working on for a big client meeting the next week. Which answer best describes your response?

A. You immediately call your boss back, thereby missing yoga class, and offer to update the spreadsheet with the latest figures, skipping lunch in the process. **(1 point)**

B. You see the text and still go into the yoga class. After yoga and a relaxing lunch, you take five minutes to double-check that your out-of-office message was securely in place. You respond to your boss's text while you're at the airport on your way home, telling him where to find the spreadsheet, and let him know that you'll be happy to discuss any updates to it on Monday morning. **(3 points)**

C. You see the text but still go to yoga. You have a hard time paying attention to your breath because your mind is preoccupied with work and wondering if you should have given clearer instructions to your team. You spend the class berating yourself for not reminding your boss (for a third time) of all the updates before you left. You convince yourself that leaving for the weekend so close to a big client meeting was a bad idea. By the end of yoga, you feel more tense than you did at the beginning of class. **(2 points)**

Question 2

It's Thanksgiving and you are invited to your in-laws' home for their yearly holiday gathering. They live across the country and air travel is exorbitant. You spend several holidays a year with this side of the family, so this is not the only chance to see them. Thanksgiving week is often packed with large group meals, activities, and events, and everyone is expected to attend. You're juggling a particularly busy workload and also have small children who are difficult to travel with. What do you do?

A. You fork out the money for airfare, spend the full week with them, and partake in all activities. You come home exhausted and behind. Your kids' routines are thrown off, and you deal with the consequences of that back home for another two weeks. **(1 point)**

B. During an argument about something completely unrelated, you bring up the Thanksgiving issue with your partner. You're pretty angry when you bring it up and quickly cut to the chase—it's not fair to spend so much time with his family over the holidays, especially during this busy year. Your partner disagrees with you, says you are overreacting. You acquiesce and end up spending the whole week there, feeling resentful, and coming home exhausted. **(2 points)**

C. Over a relaxed dinner, you bring up with your partner that you have concerns about the trip. You lay out your thoughts calmly and clearly. He disagrees with you and says that you are overreacting and should be more accommodating. You don't let it go and insist on hashing it out with him, being specific about how difficult the week will be for you, as well as the kids. After several challenging discussions, together the two of you weigh the pros and cons and decide that you will spend the money to visit but shorten the trip to four days instead of a week. **(3 points)**

Question 3

A close friend asks you to be in her wedding. It's a destination wedding and would require you to be involved in the bridal party, as well as her bridal shower and bachelorette party. In order to participate fully, you'd need to go into some debt. She is a lifelong friend and you value the relationship dearly. What do you do?

A. You say yes. As it gets closer to the wedding, you come to find out how much money will be required. You end up putting the expenses on your credit card and racking up some debt. You don't mention your financial situation to your friend, as you don't want to add stress to her big day, but internally, you feel like you've been irresponsible with your finances. **(1 point)**

B. You recognize that you don't have the money to participate fully in her wedding and know you are not willing to go into debt. But you feel too uncomfortable talking about money to bring it up with your friend. You really would like to be there for the wedding, so you say yes. However, as the event draws closer and closer, you feel more anxiety about your finances, and ultimately, you cancel a few weeks before the wedding. You feel guilt and sadness, and you've jeopardized a friendship that is important to you. **(2 points)**

C. You tell her that you're not sure what to do, as you really want to be a part of her wedding, but because of what's going on in your life, you don't have the resources to do it. She's understanding and very much wants you to be in the wedding. After a good conversation, you end up agreeing to be in the wedding party but will not be participating in the bachelorette party. You're proud of yourself for how you handled the conversation and feel like you are in a good place with your friend, despite your own feelings of disappointment for missing out on the bachelorette fun. **(3 points)**

Question 4

You've got a peripheral friend you see at group gatherings who consistently minimizes or disregards your opinion, to the point of making you feel invalidated and dismissed. What do you do?

A. You ask her out to coffee individually and talk over the situation with her by expressing what you've noticed and how it makes you feel. While the two of you never develop a super close friendship, you notice that after this conversation, she treats you with more respect. **(3 points)**

B. You say nothing, stew on it each time it happens, and wonder if you are overreacting. You spend time over text message with friends who are in different social circles analyzing this woman's behavior to see if you're in the wrong or if she is. You ultimately continue to spend time with this group, despite increasing anxiety before and after each get-together. **(1 point)**

C. You say nothing but feel increasingly distressed after each group gathering. You ultimately end up distancing yourself from that group of friends, even though you did really enjoy a good connection with other women in that circle. **(2 points)**

Question 5

You are overwhelmed by all the things in your life, and so is your partner. You'd like to find a way to have some alone time for yourself, but you feel really selfish asking for this from your partner because it means adding to their already overflowing plate as well. What do you do?

A. You avoid bringing it up because you feel like it's selfish to ask for alone time. But you feel resentful and periodically rage at them, never coming up with a realistic solution, and the quality of your relationship suffers as a result. **(1 point)**

B. You recognize that this is an issue that will only get bigger if you don't face it head-on. You bring it up in a way that encourages you both to work together to make sure you each have small amounts of alone time. You come to an agreement that every two weeks, they'll do dinner and bedtime with the kids, so you can go to your favorite yoga studio for a class. **(3 points)**

C. You bring it up with your partner and come to an agreement that it's important for you both to have some alone time. Together you make a plan for you to have one evening "off" per month. However, whenever that evening comes, you feel guilty leaving them to tend to the household and end up not taking your time away. **(2 points)**

Question 6

Your friend is in a toxic work situation. She calls you complaining about her boss and her coworkers multiple times a week. You're exhausted by her situation, which has gone on for months, and also notice that her constant complaining has not led to any action on her part. What do you do?

A. Even though texting or talking to her takes a lot of time, you say nothing, continue to take her calls, and listen to her complain a couple of times a week. You notice yourself becoming frustrated with her, but don't mention it for fear of hurting her feelings. **(1 point)**

B. You notice that a dynamic is occurring whereby you feel used by your friend. The next time she texts, you pause and take some time to respond. You tell her that you're busy that weekend and won't be able to talk, but you're not honest about the reason for distancing yourself. You feel guilt about not being there for her, and a bit stuck in the friendship, and are now avoiding her calls. **(2 points)**

C. You notice that you're spending more time giving in the relationship than she is. The next time she reaches out, you point out what you've noticed and communicate that while you support her and want to be a good friend, you cannot be her therapist or her career coach. You suggest she seek additional sources of support during this time, as you don't want this to impact the quality of your friendship in the long term. **(3 points)**

Question 7

Your parents give you unsolicited advice about a variety of important decisions in your life (e.g., whom to date, how to raise your kids, what job to take). In general, how do you respond to their advice?

A. While you wish they wouldn't offer unsolicited advice and fantasize about setting them straight, you never voice your frustration. Nine times out of ten, you follow their directives because you don't want to upset them or because you can't tolerate knowing that they disapprove of your actions. **(1 point)**

B. You're willing to consider their advice when you ask for it; however, you make your own decisions. When you decide to go in a direction that you know might cause tension, you recognize that it might cause some stress in the relationship but still move forward with your own choices. You're able to feel secure in the relationship despite knowing they disapprove. **(3 points)**

C. You feel resentful of their attempts to control your life. When you make a decision you know they would not approve of, you go to great lengths to hide your choices from them. **(2 points)**

(Score of 7–10 points) Red: You feel exhausted, overwhelmed, and constantly on edge. You find yourself daydreaming of jumping on a plane and escaping. Paradoxically, thoughts of taking time for yourself after a loaded workday, for a walk or dinner with friends, make you want to groan. The smallest request from your boss, partner, or kids has the capacity to push you into an irritable mood. When you think about how to change your situation, your mind goes blank and you just want to take a nap.

(Score of 11–17 points) Yellow: When you're yellow, you have periods of feeling overwhelmed, but you also have good periods when you feel in the driver's seat of your life. You're aware that you want to make decisions that prioritize your well-being, but you haven't figured out how to make that space for yourself. You notice that there are discrete areas in your life in which you feel run down—in your professional life, in your personal life, or with your family—but you are avoiding difficult conversations in those areas. Making decisions in your daily life feels hard, and you may experience a significant amount of guilt when making a choice that is aligned with your own values but likely to upset family, friends, or coworkers.

(Score of 18–21 points) Green: When you're green, you are thoughtfully making decisions about how you spend your time and energy. You feel like the agent of power in your life. You're able to say no despite occasionally feeling guilt. You feel generous with your time and energy, and present with your family. You have clarity in your decision-making.

Now that you've measured your real self-care level using the thermometer, don't panic if you are Red or Yellow. Setting boundaries and doing the work of real self-care is a lifelong practice. When I teach my patients about this work, I explain that real self-care is like building a muscle. It takes time to get the hang of it. Even if you are Green on the thermometer, during times of stress or in transitions you might find that you dip down to Yellow or Red.

For this reason, you will want to keep returning to a space of self-assessment and reflection. How are you doing with boundaries over time? Use the following checklist to judge your progress. Then pull it out again in a few weeks, in a few months, and as you move through the phases of your life. How is it going?

You might be Red if:

- You feel chronically overwhelmed.
- When family members, friends, or colleagues make requests, you usually don't realize you have the choice to say no.
- Small requests often make you feel irritable or angry.
- You find yourself saying yes to everything, even when you

are tired and overworked and feeling resentful after the fact (and sometimes you end up flaking out on important activities at the last minute).

- You often fantasize about dropping everything and escaping.
- You have no time for activities that help you feel better (exercise, reading your favorite books, spending quality time with friends)—*and* when you do find small amounts of time, you actively avoid these activities in favor of scrolling social media or napping.
- You rarely have the space to make deliberate decisions about how you spend your time and energy, and your life feels largely out of your control.

You might be Yellow if:

- You can say no to obligations and tasks; however, after setting a boundary you are plagued with guilt.
- You notice that the only time you don't feel guilt after setting a boundary is when someone else gives you permission to say no.
- You're aware you need to have more direct conversations with your boss or your family about division of labor or your workload—but you can't seem to bring yourself to have those talks.
- You use your vacation days and schedule alone time for yourself every so often, but as soon as you get back into your normal life, you immediately feel overworked and overwhelmed again.

You might be Green if:

- You're able to make hard decisions about how you spend your time and energy, and when guilt inevitably crops up, you don't get stuck in it.
- You recognize that it's your responsibility to communicate your needs and preferences, and more often than not, you're able to effectively do so.
- When you need to make a hard decision, you set aside time to reflect and think about your values. You recognize that it's not your job to please everyone else, and that you're doing the best you can with the resources you have available.
- You notice periods of feeling authentically generous toward others, and when this happens, you don't feel obligated.
- You don't look for permission or approval from others to make decisions about how you spend your time or energy.

Red, Yellow, or Green, we're all starting somewhere. If you're just realizing how much work you have to do, rest assured that you *can* get to Green. But like anything we want to get better at, setting boundaries requires practice and—as you'll see—some essential skills.

As you move through this chapter, reflect on the following questions:

1. When does saying no or setting boundaries come most easily for you?

2. Are there any common factors in these situations (people, places, or things)?

3. Are there situations in which it feels consistently impossible to say no or to set a boundary?

4. What supports have helped you in the past when you knew you needed and wanted to say no, and yet were hesitant to speak up?

SKILLS FOR SETTING BOUNDARIES

In this next section, I lay out four critical skills for setting boundaries. Start small, picking one skill at a time, so that you can build up your muscle. As you move through stressors and transitions in your life, return to this section, as you might find new areas that apply.

Put Guilt in the Background

My patient Tonya, thirty-nine, was newly postpartum with her first child during the pandemic and was struggling with family members who wanted to come "help" after she had her baby. Tonya and her husband both came from close-knit Jewish families who placed a strong emphasis on quality time together after the arrival of a new baby. Because her baby was born with health issues, Tonya's pediatrician had told her that they should not have any visitors who required plane travel for at least two months, as a safety precaution.

Tonya was not the least bit confused about what she wanted to do—she wanted to follow her pediatrician's recommendations. The question was whether she could give herself permission to communicate this boundary. She wondered: "Can I tolerate the guilt that will come if I set this boundary?" She knew for a fact that her mother-in-law was keen on seeing her first grandchild, and given her father-in-law's health, Tonya also knew they didn't have all the time in the world. If she said no, the guilt trip was likely to be thick. Add to this the Jewish cultural norms and the dynamics of her extended family, and Tonya felt stuck.

I frequently see women struggle with guilt tolerance, as Tonya did. Facing guilt requires accepting the fact that we cannot control and are not responsible for the emotions of other people. To effectively say no we must learn to tolerate other people's disappointment and trust that it is not a moral failing on our part. Because many of us did not develop this muscle growing up, it's not unusual for it to feel uncomfortable when we start setting boundaries as adults.

So much of the suffering I see in my practice is in women trying to "get rid of" guilt or avoid feeling guilty—they see the guilt as a giant red flag that they need to drop everything and attend to so it will go away. But this doesn't work. In trying to avoid guilt or fighting with your mind to stop feeling that way, you are still engaging with guilt and letting it (or the avoidance of it) control you. The goal is not to stop feeling guilty, but instead, to turn down the volume and not let guilt control your decisions. It means seeing the guilt not as a giant red flag but as a faulty "check en-gine" light—something that's always there but operates primarily in the background. You don't want to let it take up extra energy or have you running to the mechanic in a panic. Sure, it means *something*—but it doesn't mean everything.

In other words, guilt does not need to be our compass. It can just be a feeling in the background while we learn to reframe the discomfort as a signal that we're taking responsibility for our own emotions. As we discussed in Part I, guilt *is* pretty much always there. It comes from outside us, from the contradictory expectations that are put on women by a culture that asks us to serve others without taking up any space of our own. That feel-ing of chronic guilt is a way for women to dismiss themselves and make their own thoughts and feelings small.

When Tonya felt guilty about setting a boundary with her in-laws, she was "hooked" by the guilt. Her mind interpreted it to mean that she was in the wrong for voicing her preference. In our work together, Tonya was able to create space from her feeling of guilt using a practical strategy from acceptance and commitment therapy called *cognitive defusion*, which fosters psy-chological flexibility. *Psychological flexibility* is a clinical term that describes the capacity to develop a curious and open-ended rela-tionship with your thoughts and feelings. When you have psycho-logical flexibility, you recognize that no single thought or feeling is the capital-T truth. Cognitive defusion is a specific tech-nique to build psychological flexibility. When a difficult thought arises, instead of coming *from it*, practice looking *at it*. In essence, cognitive defusion (and, in turn, psychological flexibility) is a process of creating space between ourselves and our thoughts and feelings, so they have less power over us. It's like watching the ocean instead of being pulled by a riptide. Instead of mistaking guilt as a moral judgment on our character, we can recognize guilt for what it is: a symptom of systemic failures.

QUICK COGNITIVE DEFUSION STRATEGIES

In the same way we can set boundaries with people and situations, we can also set boundaries with our mind (i.e., our thoughts and our feelings)—and thus feel mental separation from overwhelming feelings of guilt. Like we just discussed, cognitive defusion is a strategy that effectively separates our mind from ourselves. By practicing the following thought exercises, all of which come from acceptance and commitment therapy, over time you will spend less energy fighting with your feelings of guilt and ultimately feel more confident when setting boundaries. Here are some ways to practice cognitive defusion:

Visualize the Sushi Train

The goal is not to get rid of guilt, it's to learn to coexist with it. Dr. Russ Harris, a teacher of ACT, suggests a sushi train metaphor when you are first practicing cognitive defusion. Imagine that you are in a sushi restaurant, the kind where plates of sushi are rolling out over the conveyer belt, and the chef is at the center. In this metaphor, the chef is your brain, and the plates of sushi are like the thoughts, feelings, memories, and ideas rolling through your mind all day long. When you get hooked by a thought, it's like gobbling up that piece of sushi—or stopping the conveyer belt and pushing that plate away. Instead, cognitive defusion asks you to watch the plates of sushi roll by you, without grabbing them or pushing them away.

Consider What's Workable

Instead of focusing on the *content* of the thought, focus on the *function.* Where does your guilt get you in the long run? When you stew in your guilt or make decisions in order to avoid guilt, how are your relationships impacted? Do you feel better about your workload or your family life when you let guilt lead?

Add a Catchphrase

When you find yourself spiraling into guilt or feelings of doubt after setting a boundary, try adding the phrase "My mind is telling me" in front of those guilty thoughts. Remind yourself, "There goes my mind again, telling me what to think and feel." This simple practice places some distance between yourself and your thoughts and serves to turn the volume down on the guilt.

Imagine What It Looks Like

Another strategy for gaining distance from your difficult thoughts is to give them more shape in your mind. When you hear the guilt creeping up, pause and ask yourself: "What does the guilt look like?" Does it have a color? Does it sound like someone you know? Or maybe it's a feeling in your body. For me, guilt comes in different forms—it can appear like a cloud or it can feel like nausea in my stomach. When I pinpoint and name those forms, it takes away some power from the guilty thoughts. Focusing on the form and the location of the guilt helps you separate the *thought* from *you.*

Once Tonya felt less distressed by her guilt, through her understanding and practice of cognitive defusion, she was able to communicate a clear boundary with her family and asked them to postpone their visit until several months postpartum. When the inevitable guilt trip came (which it did in full force, not just from her in-laws but also from her own parents), we practiced reframing her guilt as a feeling that was just there—an always on "check engine" light; background noise, nothing more.

Tonya recognized that she'd made the right choice for herself and her family. And later that year, when her daughter was sick and her parents stopped by (unexpected and uninvited), Tonya was able to quickly ask them to leave and refused their request to at least wake up her sleeping daughter before they left. We chalked this up as a win and a direct result of her getting comfortable tolerating her guilt. Over time, Tonya was able to recognize that the feelings of guilt were not a moral judgment on her, but instead an internalization of a lifetime of conditioning to serve everyone before herself.

Silence the Killjoys

Once you've tamed the guilt monster, the next step in setting boundaries is to recognize how other people in your life might be influencing your decisions. These people could be family members, friends, colleagues—even your church minister or a particularly memorable teacher from grade school whom you desperately wanted to impress. I refer to this group of folks whose opinions take up a disproportionate amount of space in your mind as "the killjoys."

I'm no stranger to this one. Growing up in a South Asian immigrant family, the question of "What will people say?" was ingrained into my psyche from a very young age. It wasn't until I became a psychiatrist that I understood how my fixation on controlling how other people perceive me connected to boundaries.

In my midtwenties, I found myself in a circumstance that many women go through: all of my closest friends were getting engaged and planning weddings. I was in a relationship and felt a tremendous amount of pressure from family to speed things up and to settle down with the person I was dating. At the same time, I was planning a cross-country move to start my residency in psychiatry. When I talked to my parents about the possibility of moving in with my then boyfriend without getting engaged, I was met with that familiar question: "But what will people say?" By "people," my parents meant their South Asian friends and family, as well our family in India.

I can't blame all of what followed on my parents. I was also in a rush to keep up with my friends. I did not want to be left behind, and I deemed it too costly to set a boundary with my family. I loved my boyfriend and did not want to lose him or our future together. So we got married. Ultimately, however, this chapter of my life ended in divorce, and in a tremendous amount of pain and trauma for many people I care about.

When I look back on that time now, with the twenty-twenty vision of hindsight, I see that there was a cost in the form of social capital to setting a boundary. I misjudged the cost to be too high and did not speak up for myself with the urgency that I could have out of fear of the social consequences. The problem with this mentality is that the longer you stick with a relationship, a job, or a situation that isn't working for you, the higher the emotional cost becomes to eventually set a boundary.

This personal example is admittedly an extreme version of worrying about what people will think or say, and it's one that I look back on with some shame. And to be fair, my difficulty with boundaries was not the only factor at play during this time in my life. I spent years in therapy sorting through the factors that impacted that time in my life and why I made the decisions that I did. I am sharing this story because my patients share similar ones not infrequently—situations in which the stakes are quite high and they feel ashamed for letting their fear lead—and despite being a psychiatrist, I'm not immune to these pitfalls as a human being.

As women, we are taught that others know better than us and not to trust our own intuition. We're also taught to worry more about the backlash of our decisions than to consider the risks associated with betraying ourselves. When I look back on this time in my life, I'm struck by how profoundly scared and insecure I was. I was afraid of falling out of the pack and I was terrified of losing someone I loved. In the end, both things I feared came to pass. In retrospect, the choices I made during that time were not the wrong ones for me. But because I avoided setting more firm boundaries early on, that period was much more painful and emotionally costly than it needed to be for me and for the people I cared about.

Unfortunately for me, my divorce experience didn't send me racing to embrace boundaries. (Nobody has ever accused me of being a quick study when it comes to real self-care!) My life took a vastly different direction, and I spent two years experimenting with a different lifestyle, exploring my sexuality and spirituality, and trying to understand what I wanted for myself outside the confines of my conservative South Asian parents and a rigid medical training system. As I shared during Part I, I learned some hard lessons. On one hand, I set some very firm boundaries with my family for the first time in my life and connected with what *I* wanted in life. On the other hand, I immersed myself in a high-demand group that was boundaryless because I was convinced that they had the silver bullet—the ultimate self-care practice. I was desperately looking for belonging and acceptance, and I had changed the audience from my colleagues, friends, and family to a new age group of San Francisco folks.

In the difficult aftermath of leaving that group, and with the wisdom only life experience can bring, I finally understood what I should have comprehended all along: there is no shortcut for setting boundaries and knowing your limits. The longer you let the fear of other people's judgment or reactions dictate your decisions, the more devastating the destruction is in the long run. This is precisely why boundaries are the foundation of real self-care.

You might not find yourself in situations where the stakes are so high. Maybe for you it looks like having to back out of a family trip or being viewed as the "difficult one" in your social circle. But the fear beneath setting the boundary is probably similar to what I experienced in my twenties. If you don't build this muscle of disappointing others with the little stuff, and thereby create a thicker skin to the judgment you might face, you'll end up betraying yourself when it comes to the big stuff—and you might find yourself moving forward in a relationship or in a career that isn't right for you.

So how do you let go of the worries about what the killjoys will say? First off, be wary of who you choose to listen to when it comes to boundaries. There's a maxim in psychotherapy: "Don't go to the hardware store for milk." In the context of setting healthy boundaries, this means that you should be careful about trying to get approval for setting a boundary from someone who is not capable of giving it to you. While it may be human nature to look for reassurance, sometimes those closest to us can't give it—perhaps because of patterns they learned in their own childhood or maybe because of their own inability to manage anxiety. Instead of looking externally when making tough decisions, it's critical to pay attention to your own needs and preferences.

Author and therapist Nedra Glover Tawwab, in her book *Set Boundaries, Find Peace: A Guide to Reclaiming Yourself,* says "your boundaries are a reflection of how willing you are to advocate for the life that you want."[1] She makes the important point that boundaries are not common sense, they're taught. A critical skill in setting boundaries is to separate your own needs and preferences from the opinions of other people who have a vested interest in your life.

After you've created space from the opinions and judgments of others, try "collecting data" about how different activities, relationships, and situations land in your body and work on recognizing the patterns. On one hand, which people, activities, and situations lead you to feel lighter and more expansive? Which situations or experiences leave you feeling more energetic than when you started? These physical signals steer you toward saying yes. On the other hand, which people, activities, and situations cause your body to tighten up, give you a feeling of dread, palpitations, or even nausea? This is your body saying no. When someone approaches you with a request and you don't have any of these physical responses, it's a signal to ask questions, like "What's the deadline for this project?" or "Who else is coming to the party?" Get clarification and pay attention to how your body feels when you receive answers. Accordingly, you can then say yes or no, depending on the information you learn.

Ultimately, the understandable fear that we all have when setting boundaries is linked to whether it is emotionally safe to express our truth or whether people will reject us. Depending on the type of family in which you grew up, this fear can be more pronounced. My patients who grew up in critical environments have a more difficult time feeling safe enough in their relationships to exert a boundary. This is because it can sometimes feel like saying no or stating a preference will cause a break in the relationship. And the reality is, in unhealthy relationships, these breaks *do* happen.

Families in which there is addiction or trauma also often lack boundaries; in these family systems there is usually one person, either the addict or the abusive individual, who dictates how the group reacts. Family members who attempt to set boundaries will be judged, criticized, or even abused.[2]

Cultural components come into play as well, and I experienced this myself as a South Asian. Immigrant families may balk at boundary-setting because non-Western cultures tend to adopt a more communal mentality toward decision-making. If you grew up in a family where you never saw adults have open conversations about their decision-making and the expectation was for each member of the family to acquiesce to the larger group's needs, it may be more difficult for you to make these choices for yourself now.

Healthy adult relationships should be able to accommodate the needs and preferences of each person. In a healthy relationship—whether between two partners, extended family members, or even coworkers—boundaries are a way of putting *more* of yourself into your relationships, because you are sharing your needs and your preferences. In Chapter 7, we will cover how to identify your values, which are what you can use to guide your decisions instead of guilt or worry about judgment from others.

To Practice: Putting the Self Back in Self-Care

The way others react to our decisions when we set a boundary or negotiate is a powerful Rorschach test. A Rorschach test is an old-time Freudian tool psychiatrists and psychologists used to analyze their patients' personality traits. Basically, the way someone else reacts to your boundaries tells us more about *them* than it does about you. If you find yourself focusing your attention on what the killjoys think and want, as opposed to what *you* think and want, this exercise will help you reframe the running mantra of "What will people think?"

1. Think about the last time you either wanted to say no to a request or had follow-up questions to a request and worried about how those questions would be received.
2. Now visualize the people in your life who would be upset with you, and instead of focusing on their negative feelings, reflect on what their anger tells you about them. Think about what their reaction says about their view of the world, your role in their life, and their unspoken expectations.

Visualizing and reflecting on what these reactions tell you about folks is a powerful way to remind yourself that others bring their own opinions and life experiences into their interactions with you. Turning the focus on their unique history and context gives you more space to make decisions that work for you.

Know Your Three Choices

Setting healthy boundaries isn't just about learning to say no. It's also about making clear and concise requests of others, and this too is a key component of real self-care. In all situations, you have three choices: you can say yes, you can say no, or you can negotiate. This decision-making framework builds on the previous point that your boundary is in your pause. When you take the time to consider all the options and reflect on the potential risks and benefits of saying yes or saying no, you are exerting a boundary. The third option—negotiating—means asking questions, gathering information, and making requests before saying yes or saying no.

For my patient Tonya, whom we met earlier in this chapter, the skill of negotiation came up when planning for a summer vacation. For the past five years, her partner's family would rent an Airbnb at a nearby lake, and spend two weeks boating, fishing, and enjoying outdoor sports. This particular summer, Tonya was two months postpartum and they also had a very active toddler. Her in-laws assumed that Tonya and her husband would participate fully like in previous years.

Because she had been actively working on real self-care, Tonya recognized that she had choices. On one hand, driving for three hours with a two-month-old seemed daunting. She was also worried about safety precautions for her toddler during water sports and what type of activities would be on the agenda. On the other hand, she did enjoy the summer visits to the lake, and recognized that it could be a nice break for her to have extra hands to help take care of the baby. Instead of immediately saying yes, like she normally would have, Tonya told her mother-in-law that she would get back to her. She asked questions about the plans for the lake trip, including about how much room there would be, the sleeping arrangements, and the safety precautions for the house they had rented. In the end, Tonya and her partner decided to visit for one week instead of two, and Tonya felt proud of herself for how she had handled the situation.

My patient Angela, whom you met at the beginning of the chapter, also embraced the skill of negotiating in her relationship. In our work together, we noticed Angela had a habit of quickly accommodating her boyfriend's requests, even at the cost of goals that were important to her—such as her performance in her master's program. Despite living together, and both working full-time jobs, Angela hesitated to turn over household tasks to her boyfriend.

In a session one day, as we were talking about her avoidance of negotiations around dividing chores, Angela said, "Honestly, isn't it just easier for me to do things by myself? The work of saying no or negotiating feels like it's just another burden that falls on my shoulders, and then I'm stuck dealing with the backlash from everyone in my life."

Angela had a fair point. She'd had varying degrees of success with getting her partner to pull his weight in managing household tasks. It certainly did create more work on her part to try to hold him accountable.

While boundaries themselves are not cocreated, the work of communicating them and coming to a solution is very much a negotiation between people. It also requires more invisible labor that falls on the shoulders of women. Not only is negotiating more work, it's also emotionally messy—you have to wait to see if the other person will come around, and you have to trust that your requests are reasonable, despite pushback from others.

When it comes to boundaries, though, we are training the people in our lives how to treat us with our words, decisions, and actions. When we verbalize a clear boundary, it helps other people understand how we expect them to behave, and in the long run, this *saves* time. Eve Rodsky, author of *Fair Play: A Game-Changing Solution for When You Have Too Much to Do (and More Life to Live)*, describes what she calls the "Toxic Time Message: I can save time by doing it myself."[3] She explains how common it is for women, who bear the heavy mental load of household CEO, to mistakenly believe that it's smarter and easier for them to get all the little tasks done because their partners are less efficient and never get them done quite right. What these women don't calculate is the resentment and rage that build up over years and years of just doing it all because it's "easier and faster." It may seem easier to do it all in the short term, but when it comes to boundaries, we need to be in it for the long haul. The goal is a system that operates through the work of multiple adults—not just you.

With time, Angela was able to recognize how her need for

expediency and her impatience with her boyfriend's methodology (or lack thereof) for cleaning the kitchen had her focused on the short term, instead of the implications for their relationship. She also learned how to tolerate the uncertainty involved in waiting for him to restock the toilet paper, instead of rushing to handle it herself. Together, she and her boyfriend were able to navigate shared household responsibilities, which ultimately led her to feel better about moving forward in the relationship with him.

Clearly Communicate Your Boundaries

Once you've started working on what gets in the way of setting boundaries, you can then begin communicating your choices to friends, family, and colleagues. My advice here is to start small and pick low-stakes situations in the beginning. It can be helpful to use scripts when you are starting out, so I've included some here, along with helpful communication tips to use as a guide.

Be Clear

When stating a boundary, it's not the time for wishy-washy language. Instead, you want to be direct and firm. For example, instead of "I was wondering if you still need that client report back by the end of this week?" say, "Is the priority the expense report or the client report? I will not be able to complete both by Friday, so please let me know where I should focus my attention."

Don't Ask for Permission

Boundaries aren't cocreated. Remember that you're the one making the decision, and the other person is allowed to have their reaction. You can express that it was a difficult decision to make and that you put a lot of thought into it, but you should steer clear of asking for permission. Instead of saying, "Is it okay if we talk later?" say, "I'm not able to talk this weekend. I'll call you next week."

Try Not to Overexplain

It's helpful to be concise with your boundary—whether it's starting with a clear "I'm afraid that doesn't work for me," or asking for clarifying information ("When will you need that back by?"). When you go on too long, trying to explain your decision to someone, it can come across as trying to ask for permission.

It's Okay to Use Email If Needed

If you find yourself easily backtracking on the phone, or if text messaging leads to heated threads, email can be a nice substitute. It gives you time to compose your thoughts and lends itself to a more measured response.

Some of my favorite scripts for saying no and making requests are on the next pages. I consider it a productive week when I have used one of them at least three times.

"I wish I could swing it, but I'm swamped. Can we check in next month?"

"I appreciate you thinking of me for this role, but I'm prioritizing ———— at the moment. I'd be happy to consider this next year."

"My schedule has changed. Can we please reschedule this meeting for ————?"

"I'll need your help with ————. Can you please be home by ———— tonight?"

"No, I'm not free to talk right now."

"I notice that ———— isn't working. Can we set aside some time to discuss it?"

Of note, depending on the culture you come from and even the area of the country that you live in, you may need to adapt these scripts to fit your needs. If you come from a culture that values communality and interdependency, it can be more difficult to set boundaries. In these circumstances it can be helpful to work with a therapist who is knowledgeable about your culture and who can help you tease apart the implications of setting boundaries. At the end of the book, I've included a resource list for finding professional help.

WHEN TO SEEK PROFESSIONAL HELP

Clinical depression and anxiety both make it difficult to set effective boundaries with people who are close to us. These conditions impact our brain's ability to cope with difficult emotions. Thus, someone with major depressive disorder is going to feel and internalize the guilt trip coming from extended family more powerfully than someone without major depressive disorder. And someone with clinical anxiety—like generalized anxiety disorder or obsessive-compulsive disorder—is going to have a more difficult time letting go of control. If you notice a pattern of being unable to set boundaries or consistently backtracking on them, working with a mental health professional can be crucial.

Like I mentioned earlier, there is a little bit of chicken and egg going on when it comes to real self-care and clinical mental health conditions. On one hand, having a clinical mental health condition makes it more difficult to do the work of real self-care, because your nervous system is not functioning optimally and you will have a harder time dealing with the backlash from family and friends. On the other hand, if you struggle with a mental health condition, you can use your real self-care practice as a barometer of sorts. If you're finding that you're able to set boundaries and effectively deal with guilt, that can be an indicator that you're doing well. When setting boundaries falls by the wayside and you are spending more of your time ruminating on guilty thoughts, that can be a sign that your mental health is worsening.

The following situations indicate you would benefit from seeing a mental health professional:

- The backlash you receive from family and friends leads you to experience very low lows. You have feelings that you'd be better off not existing or that life isn't worth living, and your functioning is impacted. You have to call in sick to work because you can't get out of bed.

- Your avoidance of setting boundaries has led you to live in a constant state of unease, to the point where you are having panic attacks or extreme bouts of anxiety.

- You find yourself constantly preventing other people from stepping in and helping out with tasks—large or small. It's very difficult for you to watch someone complete a chore if it's not done to your exact specifications. Your inability to accept help or to delegate tasks has caused problems in your relationships or has led to symptoms of a mental health condition.

- You consistently find yourself seeking reassurance or approval from people in your life who cannot give it to you, and you become upset when their advice feels critical or hurtful.

- It's impossible for you to tease out on your own which people, situations, or activities you genuinely enjoy and which people, situations, or activities you dread.

By now I hope you've seen how setting boundaries is like building a new set of muscles. It will feel uncomfortable at first, but as you train, you build up strength, and it gets easier to have these conversations. I recommend starting out small and letting go of lower-stakes tasks—perhaps rescheduling an item on your calendar or bowing out of a social event. By beginning this way, you'll come to see that even a tiny shift goes a long way. Use the framework of cultivating psychological flexibility, recognize the costs of focusing on what other people think, and proactively ask questions and make requests as you move along. Over time you'll find that you can make weightier decisions more easily. Every boundary you set is a reminder that you have agency over how you spend your time and your energy.

SOUNDS GREAT, BUT . . .

Maybe all that I've put forth in this chapter sounds great to you in theory, but you're still unsure of how this comes together in practice. In each chapter going forward, the "Sounds Great, but . . ." section will address common questions and ways to handle tough situations.

I would love to be able to say no to some of the responsibilities on my plate, but I'm the primary breadwinner in my home, I have a special-needs son, and my parents rely on me for social and financial support. I don't feel like I have the option to say no, or even to negotiate. Literally everything on my plate feels critical, and if I drop the ball on something, the health of people I love (my son, my parents) will suffer.

The author Nora Roberts was asked how she could possibly juggle her work, her family life, her own mental health, and so on when she must have had five gazillion balls in the air. Nora's famous response was that the key to staying afloat was recognizing which of these balls were rubber and which were made of glass. You'll need to drop some, but you want to make sure the ones that drop are rubber. It's a great line, but it raises a question—what if all the balls feel like glass?

If you're in an impossible situation like this one, keep in mind the following: First, you're allowed to be angry—you're allowed to rage at the system. Feeling this anger is important, and it helps to have others in your corner who will validate that rage. Our system is not set up fairly, especially for a woman who is serving as a caregiver. (I've got lots more to say about channeling this rage—see Chapter 6.)

After you've raged, the next step is to figure out if, inside this impossible situation, there are actually any small spaces where you can let go of something tiny on your plate, wherein the consequences are less severe and perhaps some of these balls that seem like glass are in reality made of rubber. To make this assessment, you'll need to set aside a discrete period of time when your nervous system is not in panic mode. (When you're in panic mode, everything feels dire and you can't make rational determinations about whether a ball is glass or rubber.) In this calm space, reflect honestly and realistically about whether the pace at which you are going is sustainable. What would life look like three months from now, six months from now, if you let a couple of balls drop? For example, when faced with a looming work deadline and a family member unexpectedly falls ill and needs your help, can you explain your situation to your boss and see if there is flexibility in the schedule? Or instead of going all-out and accounting for the preferences of each extended family member when preparing to host a holiday dinner, could you set a limit on how much time and energy you will spend on preparation, regardless of the opinions of the killjoys?

Most of my patients, when they step back and allow themselves to think about the future, recognize that something has to give. It cannot be a long-term or sustainable solution to go at two hundred miles an hour and/or be a caretaker for your loved ones while your own health gets worse. Like we discussed, the key to change is taking small steps. Experiment with micro changes and see what it feels like. It can also be helpful to sit down with a trusted friend, list everything you do each day, and bounce ideas off them for tasks that you can let go of or where you can take shortcuts. Even when—to be frank, *especially* when—the health and well-being of your dependents rests on your shoulders, you still need time for yourself. To borrow Nora's metaphor, if you don't let some of the rubber balls drop once in a while, eventually the glass balls will start dropping too.

I'm a Black woman, and my job provides benefits for my whole family. If I were to lose my job, the impact would be devastating. I'm called upon to do a lot of invisible labor in the office, such as coordinating schedules and organizing birthday parties, and am asked to partake in it more than my white colleagues. I am deeply resentful of this unpaid labor. But I'm worried that if I speak up about my boundaries, I will be labeled the angry Black woman, and I will be pushed out. How do I set a boundary when the stakes are so high for me and for my family?

I spoke with my friend and colleague Kali Cyrus, MD, a psychiatrist and an expert in managing conflicts stemming from diversity and difference. Dr. Cyrus, a queer Black woman, has personally dealt with overt racism and discrimination, as well as microaggressions in the workplace. She helps her patients navigate working in systems where their labor and their humanity are not valued.

For many women, especially those living in poverty and Black women, the line between swimming and sinking is thin. But, Dr. Cyrus asks, what if in some situations, on that edge between sinking and swimming, there is an opportunity? She says, "It is almost like the perceived injustice is so clear, and instead of just resulting in rage and powerlessness, there is a sense of empowerment. You end up confronting your boss, or writing that email, or speaking up for yourself." In other words, sometimes the emotional labor that you must do in order to keep up with the status quo of a toxic environment becomes so high that the scale shifts, and you notice yourself feeling ready to push back, despite the costs that may come.

In these situations, the best way to assess the risks involved with setting boundaries is to say no to a small task and then monitor the results closely. In parallel, you can also come up with a plan ahead of time in case your boundary setting leads to adverse consequences—this might mean polishing your résumé or beginning to network with colleagues in your industry. If setting even a small limit leads to a reprimand, that's a powerful data point about whether it's healthy for you to stay in this setting in the long run.

Okay, I love the idea of setting boundaries, but I have so many commitments on my plate that I've already said yes to. There are people depending on me, and I don't want to let them down. I understand saying no to new things, but aren't I a quitter if I back out of these commitments?

I hear you. It's a lot easier to say no to what's incoming than to clean up shop inside the house. But I'll share a catchy mantra I learned from actress Tabitha Brown: "*I changed my mind* is a full sentence." In the complicated world we live in, our situations are constantly changing and becoming more complex. It's unrealistic and unforgiving to expect that you will never need to make changes to your commitments.

I recommend keeping a running log of your activities—personal, work, and family-related—and every three months, reevaluating which items provide value and which no longer fit your life. In Chapter 7 we will be talking about identifying values and how this helps us decide where we spend our time, so keep reading for more guidance about making these decisions.

For now, remember that you can only fully enjoy the good *new* things in your life if you are making space by clearing out the obligations that no longer serve you. Maybe that's a friendship you've outgrown or an extra work project that you're not getting paid for. Whatever it is, it's okay to let it go even if you said yes in the past.

THE BOUNDARIES BULLETIN

Your quick list when it comes to boundaries

- Your boundary is in your *pause*—you can say yes, you can say no, or you can negotiate.

- When communicating boundaries, be clear, be concise, and don't apologize.

- The point of setting a boundary is to communicate what *you* need in a relationship—not to control the other person's response.

- Just because you feel guilt does not mean you are making the wrong choice. Guilt does not need to be your compass.

- Don't go to the hardware store for milk (i.e., be careful about trying to get approval for setting a boundary from someone who is not capable of giving it to you).

- You are allowed to change your mind.

- If you've never set boundaries in the past, it's normal for it to feel uncomfortable.

- Start small and build your boundaries muscle over time.

Chapter 6

REAL SELF-CARE MEANS TREATING YOURSELF WITH COMPASSION

PERMISSION TO BE GOOD ENOUGH

Remember that self-love is also revolutionary and world changing.

AMANDA GORMAN

A few years ago, I was teaching a moms' group to support postpartum mental health. One new mom, attending with her newborn daughter, reported that so far, her postpartum period was going well, and she was enjoying motherhood more than she had expected. Her question to the group was about maternity leave: her employer offered her an unexpected *extra* two weeks of paid leave. She wasn't sure what to do. If she said yes, she would be leaving surprise work for her already overburdened team, and that made her feel guilty. If she said no, she would be missing a precious two weeks with her daughter, and that felt bad too. What should she do? I asked her if there was *any* solution about which she would not beat herself up. That got her attention. It had never occurred to her that in the face of an unexpected opportunity, her mind had created a narrative that could *only* end in bad feelings for herself.

For women, beating ourselves up is practically second nature. Regardless of what choice this new mother made, in her mind it had been decided that she was failing. The concept that she was a person worthy of trust, goodwill, and compassion was remarkably foreign.

As we discussed in the previous chapter, learning to set boundaries and deal with the inevitable guilt that comes afterward is the backbone to real self-care. However, the work doesn't end there. Rather, you build on it to access the second principle of real self-care: treating yourself with compassion.

First, let's get clear on the definition of self-compassion. You may have some preconceived notions about what self-compassion is, and they may or may not include a massage in a crystal-filled room or a "treat yourself" mentality. Or maybe you hear the phrase *self-compassion* and want to run for the hills. Confession—I was in the latter category. Despite attending years of therapy, self-compassion as I imagined it had always felt weak to me—I felt like I was giving myself a fake pep talk while not believing a word I was saying.

But there's a different way to think about self-compassion, one that focuses on your relationship with your mind and is grounded in psychological flexibility. This is the type of self-compassion I'm talking about here. When you're struggling with cruel self-talk, this psychological self-compassion is exactly the salve you need.

Kristin Neff, PhD, one of the foremost researchers on self-compassion, divides the skill into three components:

1. Replacing self-judgment with self-kindness
2. Recognizing your shared humanity
3. Being curious about negative thoughts instead of believing them as the immediate truth (psychological flexibility again)

Dr. Neff also draws a clear distinction between self-compassion and self-esteem. While self-esteem builds up our psychological defense by cultivating a feeling of high self-regard, self-compassion is a method for developing self-clarity. For example, while "I'm the youngest attorney to make partner in my firm's history, so I must be doing something right" might help with self-esteem, self-compassion asks us to look inward and reflect on how we treat ourselves. It looks more like: "I felt scared while going up for partner, and I took care of myself with kindness."

Research shows that people who cultivate self-compassion are more likely to be proactive in making positive changes in their lives, like being assertive in their choices.[1] One study of almost seven hundred mothers showed that women with higher levels of self-compassion had fewer negative thoughts and a less judgmental view of themselves.[2] That sounds like a healthy place from which to do the real work of self-care, doesn't it?

Real self-care requires treating yourself with humanity and being in tune with what you need and want at any given moment.

And so, when you're practicing real self-care, self-compassion is the lens through which you view yourself. It's about recognizing your shortcomings or the ways in which life doesn't match your expectations, and instead of taking out the boxing gloves, offering yourself a dose of kindness.

What I've found most helpful is to take a close look at the way I talk to myself when things are going wrong. When I inevitably end up criticizing myself, I practice substituting harsh and critical language with more kind and flexible thinking. I call this *setting boundaries with myself*. This is another way to develop psychological flexibility, which we discussed in Chapter 5.

While I was writing this book, the need for self-compassion came up front and center in my life in an utterly powerful and personal way. My life partner, Justin, and I were going through the IVF process to start our family together. Assisted reproductive technology is a juggernaut of doctor appointments, blood draws, at-home injection medications, and calendars timed down to the minute. To say I was overwhelmed was an understatement. I noticed myself teetering between two opposite extremes. Double- and triple-checking the doses of all of my medications and managing my doctor's visits meant that, ultimately, the success of this process and whether we could have a baby rested completely on my shoulders—I'd better not mess this up. And yet, on the complete opposite side, I knew that I was a thirty-seven-year-old woman whose body and reproductive system was going to do what it was going to do. Whether reproductive science worked for me and my partner really was not in our hands—we had to have faith in our doctor, team, the process, and ourselves. Not only did I need to embrace the dialectic, I also had to develop compassion for myself.

For me, that meant setting boundaries for how much self-deprivation I would endure. I put a limit on how much googling I did, and how many friends and colleagues I spoke to about the science of IVF. I decided not to go on any of the extreme fertility diets, but I cut out caffeine and alcohol (not fun!). I told myself, over and over again—"I am enough" and "I am doing enough." In this process, I could not control the outcome, but what I could control was how I treated myself—mentally and physically. As much as this whole ethos of self-kindness goes against my personality, I forced myself (definitely kicking and screaming) to be kind.

TAMING MARTYR MODE

Before we dive into the tools of how to practice compassion toward ourselves, there is an important barrier to self-compassion that we must first address—Martyr Mode. Martyr Mode occurs when you find yourself taking care of everyone and everything around you, only to find yourself burnt to a crisp. We saw this earlier with Mikaleh, who was single-parenting two daughters and taking care of her sick father. Mikaleh felt *pride* about how much she worried about and did for her family. On one hand, being a martyr is about experiencing suffering and destroying yourself for the sake of others, whether it's your children, family, or even your coworkers. On the other hand, it's about relishing your sacrifice and, paradoxically, making sure that your smallness is seen. Women get a ton of social approval for self-sacrificing and making ourselves smaller and smaller. With Martyr Mode, there can be a particular self-satisfaction that comes when you save the day and take one for the team.

We all know these people (and maybe we've been them). They are the ones who want you to know how long they slaved over the stove, only to brush off any compliments. Or the ones who seem to be competing with you in their suffering—"You worked fifty hours last week? Well did you know I keep a sleeping bag under my desk so I can spend the night in the office?"

It begs the question: What is this race we are competing in, and who wins here?

The problem is, when we engage in Martyr Mode, we are falling into a behavior pattern without first being willing to offer compassion to ourselves. *We mistakenly believe compassion will come from the outside, if only we earn it by serving others.*

I've been there myself—let me share one example. After about a year of the IVF process, I was fortunate to get pregnant. This in itself was certainly happy and relieving news because I had previously suffered a miscarriage. But as I moved into the third trimester of my pregnancy, it was as if a switch flipped in my mind—all of a sudden my Martyr Mode kicked into high gear. I was preparing my patients for my upcoming maternity leave, I had a looming book deadline, my company, Gemma, was launching a new product—and there would soon be a baby to take care of! I watched myself become resentful: Didn't everyone else know just *how much* I needed to get done? Why weren't they all stepping in to help me?

On one occasion, I got snippy with my team, and my cofounder called me out (lovingly). I was treating myself like a martyr and everyone else around me could see it, loud and clear. I recognized what was going on, and using the tools that I share with you over the next pages, I was able to establish a reconnection with my inner self-compassionate voice. I hope my personal experience helps you understand that, like all real self-care, developing self-compassion is not one and done. With every transition in life, we will have to reorient ourselves. The reassuring news is once you learn these skills, they are always available for you to turn to in times of transition and stress.

How do you know if you're falling into Martyr Mode? A telltale sign is when you extend yourself toward others and have an unspoken expectation that something—praise, support, attention—will be given in return. When that expectation is not met, you lose your cool and are secretly (or rather not so secretly) seething.

Falling into the Martyr Mode trap doesn't always correlate to a clinical diagnosis; it's a role women can inhabit while also being highly functioning and excelling in their lives. On the inside, however, when a woman is stuck in Martyr Mode, she has convinced herself that the best way to make choices is to put herself last. Martyr Mode makes it feel like life is happening to you, as opposed to you being the agent of your own life.

It's the polar opposite of real self-care.

This phenomenon doesn't only apply to mothers. Women and girls in our culture are socially conditioned to give their time, energy, and attention to others, whether that's in the home or the workplace. Girls are praised in the classroom and on the playground for being nice and yielding to their peers. Fast-forward a decade or two, and women are the ones ordering the birthday cakes and on the (unpaid) mentorship committees. It's not that these acts of service are bad—what's wrong is the assumption that women will take them on *and*, in the process, put their own needs second.

All of this said, we come by Martyr Mode honestly. When we are operating in Martyr Mode, we hope to control the reactions and responses of our would-be critics. And because we live in a culture that loves to penalize women for setting boundaries and claiming space for themselves, this makes sense as a defense mechanism. Think about that time your house looked like a tornado had just blown through and you decided to take a nap instead of clean, only to have your mom stop by and snarkily comment how nice it is that you can "take it easy" with dirty dishes in the sink. Thanks, Mom! Or think about the woman who gets berated on social media for choosing a child-free life. Or the woman who gets ridiculed for leaving the paid workforce to raise her family. No matter what choice we make, as Martha Beck reminds us, the modern woman's dilemma is a riddle that defies logic, and the critics are many and loud.[3]

The first and most important step of self-compassion is giving yourself permission to practice it. I hope it's now clear to you why we must let go of Martyr Mode to take that first step. Giving yourself permission to practice self-compassion is, in and of itself, an act of compassion.

As you move through this chapter, reflect on the following questions:

- In what situations is it relatively easy for you to speak kindly to yourself?
- Are there any common factors in these situations (people, places, or things)?
- Are there people, places, or things that consistently make it difficult to treat yourself with compassion or situations in which your self-criticism is extraordinarily loud?
- When you find yourself engaged in Martyr Mode, reflect on what gifts (in terms of attention, help, or energy) you are expecting to get paid back with, even if those expectations are beneath the surface.
- Name one situation in which you were surprised or caught off guard by the kindness or generosity you gave to yourself. Reflect on the circumstances that allowed for your self-compassion.

Self-compassion is easier for me to understand and implement if I think of it as a new way to work with my brain. This way, it's less about "going easy on myself" and more about paying attention to how I talk to myself and slowly learning a new language.

In the following pages, I'll share with you the tools that I have found most useful for nurturing a self-compassionate frame of mind.

ADD "OUCH!" TO YOUR VOCABULARY

My patient Sonia, a Muslim American woman in her midthirties, came to see me for treatment of her lifelong depression. Over the course of our work together, she had two children, while also being employed full time outside the home in advertising. Like most mothers in America, she struggled with balancing All the Things, and when the going got tough, she beat herself up. One day in a therapy session, after deciding to send both of her sons to their babysitter for a Sunday afternoon (so that she could catch up on work), Sonia said, "Jeez, I can't believe I'm shipping my kids off to a babysitter. Why did I even have kids if I was just going to send them off for someone else to take care of even on the weekend?"

My response was an immediate and visceral "Ouch."

Sonia looked up, surprised, and said, "Huh? What do you mean?"

"That's really mean," I said. "Do you always talk to yourself like that? Would you say something like that to a friend?"

She stopped and considered her frame of mind. She agreed that not only was she being quite cruel to herself, she would also never speak to a friend like that.

In our work together, we came to uncover that Sonia's inner critic—the voice in her head that criticized and judged her every action—was actually the voice of her mother. Growing up, Sonia had internalized her mother's voice, and now it sounded quite like her own. It was difficult at first for Sonia to pick up on her inner critic, but once we started to spot it, she noticed it every single time she made a decision in service of real self-care. It was like clockwork.

Note that inner critics are not all bad. Maybe your inner critic got you through a tough childhood or traumatic circumstances. You can simultaneously be grateful for your fierce inner critic and how she protected you through difficult times earlier in life, while also recognizing that her tough-as-nails approach no longer serves you in the same way.

To Practice: Naming Your Inner Critic

Acceptance and commitment therapy teaches that one of the best ways to gain awareness around how you talk to yourself is to dial in to your inner critic. Pay attention to what the voice looks and feels like. For many of us, inner critics are the voices of people who were an instrumental force in our childhood. However, in order to take some of the power out of that voice, as an adult, you can rename it.

For one week, keep track of the words and phrases that your inner critic uses to make you feel bad. Write down the exact phrases that come up, no matter how harsh they sound. After you've got your notes, come up with a popular cultural stand-in that represents your inner critic. I'll go first. My inner critic is

Angelica, from the kids' cartoon *Rugrats*. She's bossy, she's a know-it-all, and she loves to see you fail. A patient of mine named her inner critic Miranda Priestly, the terrifying Anna Wintour–type character from *The Devil Wears Prada*.

By putting some drama into your inner critic, you lighten up the voice and remind yourself that this critic isn't your own voice—instead it's an amalgamation of the worst killjoys you can imagine. It's much easier to say, "Ouch," to that voice when it's Anna Wintour or Angelica than when it feels like your own.

DIAL DOWN THE SHAME

We can't talk about inner critics or the impact of Martyr Mode without tackling the powerful feeling of shame. Shame is the belief that we are inherently unworthy, wrong, or bad. When self-compassion feels impossible, shame is typically lurking beneath the surface. Brené Brown points out that shame shows up in two main forms in our minds:

- "You are never good enough."
- "Who do you think you are?"[4]

Shame is a different emotion than guilt. We feel guilt when we believe we've made a mistake—taken the wrong course of action, hurt someone, or committed an offense. Shame, on the other hand, isn't specific to any one action or decision. Shame occurs when you feel wrong as a whole person. It's a feeling of otherness or of not belonging. One mom might feel *guilty* because she yelled at her kids, for instance, but another mom might feel *shame* because she is a "bad mom" for yelling at her kids.

All of us have periods when we fall into shame-based thinking. It can be tempting to get down on yourself for this, but the goal of self-compassion is to lighten your shame, not to increase it, and I don't want you beating yourself up even more than you already do.

That said, you do need to recognize it. When we talk to ourselves from a shame-based point of view, it looks like what Sonia did, berating herself for sending her kids to the babysitter so she could get some work done on a Sunday. You can practically see the big neon lights screaming WHO DO YOU THINK YOU ARE? above Sonia's head, right? It's pretty much the polar opposite of self-compassion. And when we let that shame-based voice win, Martyr Mode kicks into high gear, our inner critic goes wild, and we end up constructing situations in which it's impossible for us to feel good. When this happens, we start from a place of "wrong" or of failure, instead of starting from a place of acceptance and kindness. So, logically, the antidote to shame-based self-talk is to first notice when it is happening, and second, to inject a reminder that you are Good Enough.

The term *good enough* comes from the psychological concept of "the Good Enough mother," which was coined by Dr. Donald Winnicott, an English pediatrician and psychoanalyst. This concept proposes that the role of a parent is to provide their child with a background environment that allows the child to develop the ability to tolerate their own distress.[5] The Good Enough mother does not jump at every cry or startle. Instead, she allows her child to feel slight frustration as he learns his way in the world. In the context of developing self-compassion for ourselves, I am asking you to come from a mental framework of Good Enough, as opposed to a shame-based internal narrative. Coming from Good Enough means that you acknowledge your humanity and give yourself the generosity that you would extend to others. You trust that the people you care about can tolerate small discomforts and mistakes.

Here's what coming from Good Enough means to me:

- I am okay with making mistakes. (*I don't need to listen to the cruel voice in my head.*)
- I am not defined by being selfish or selfless. (*I am allowed to consider myself along with those who I care about when I make decisions.*)
- I can extend the compassion I give to others to myself. (*I believe that we all deserve compassion, myself included.*)

To Practice: Coming from Good Enough

If you are coming from a shame-based mentality, you might be held back by worries about being selfish, and instead of choosing real self-care, you might swing closer to selfless (and thus Martyr Mode). Accessing Good Enough means that you are finding a middle ground between selfish and selfless. This exercise will give you a taste of how coming from a starting assumption of Good Enough feels different.

1. Think of a recent situation in which your needs and preferences were in conflict with those who are close to you or whom you are responsible for. It might have been in relation to your paid work, or maybe it was at home with your partner or your family. You might remember a Martyr Mode feeling of anger or resentment.

2. Now imagine this situation, but first start with the assumption that you handled it by being selfish. What choice would the "selfish" version of you make? What were the reasons that "selfish you" had for making that choice? How did others react to your decision? How did you feel afterward?

3. Imagine the situation a second time, starting with the assumption that you handled it by being selfless. What choice would the "selfless" version of you make? What were the reasons that "selfless you" had for this choice? How did others react to your decision? How did you feel afterward?

4. Now reimagine the situation for a final time but start with the assumption that you are Good Enough. When you come from Good Enough, you are approaching your decision by wanting the best for all parties, including yourself, and you are valuing the feelings, time, and energy of everyone equally. What choice did you make? How did others react?

How did making this decision feel different than the first two examples?

When considering how it feels to make your decision from a position of Good Enough, keep in mind the following:

- How does my fear of being selfish prevent me from accessing Good Enough?
- What are the costs (physical, emotional, spiritual) of being selfless?
- In which areas of my life do I feel most convinced of being Good Enough? Can I bring the conviction that I am Good Enough to other areas of my life, in which I am less certain of my inherent Good Enough quality?

You are the only one who can give yourself the permission of starting from Good Enough. Be careful about getting caught up in wishful thinking that other people in your life will gift you this skill; self-compassion cannot be air-dropped—you have to build it yourself. By cultivating a mindset of Good Enough, you will naturally bring more compassion into your internal narrative.

DISTINGUISH BETWEEN YOUR CRITIC AND YOUR DRIVE

You might find yourself thinking, "But wait, isn't my inner critic what helps me be a productive, functioning adult? If I didn't have an inner critic, would I ever be on time again? Could I hold down a job?" How do you keep *drive* without a *critic*, and where does the line get crossed?

Our goal with self-compassion is not to eliminate the inner critic but instead to recognize when it's become too harsh and when it is serving in a counterproductive way. Instead of arguing with or trying to eliminate the inner critic, remember that it's just one voice in our minds, in a sea of other ideas, thoughts, and feelings. The problem is not that the critic exists; the problem is when it's the only or loudest voice, because it leads to counterproductive feelings and thoughts. When your inner critic is loudest, you get sapped of your energy—joy and meaning leave you, and you're simply going through the motions.

For example, when Angelica of *Rugrats* infamy was berating me for not getting more writing done, the last thing I wanted to do was sit down and write about real self-care. Not only did I feel like a hypocrite, I also couldn't hear myself think clearly. Paradoxically, when I gave myself permission to take the night off, go for a walk, or listen to my favorite podcast episode, I felt inspired to write.

Let's take the simple example of being on time. When you find yourself running late for a party, what does your inner voice sound like?

- Option 1: "Hey, loser, you're definitely going to be late again. Your friends are so fed up with you! Why did you even agree to go in the first place?"

- Option 2: "Remember that it always takes ten extra minutes in traffic, so stop fussing with your makeup because you don't want to be late. Everyone is so excited to hear about how your first art show went!"

What's baked into Option 1 is "I'm a bad person." If your voice sounds more like Option 1, your job is to set boundaries with the inner critic and come from a place of assuming Good Enough intent instead of a shame-based place. Can you find a voice that sounds more like Option 2? Can you remember why you want to be at this party?

If you don't learn how to speak to yourself with respect, kindness, and nurturing, then when you arrive at your destination—whether that is finishing writing a book or showing up at a friend's party—you will be on your last legs. You don't *need* to have a cruel inner critic to get things done. The only reason so many of us think we do is because we have become habituated to that voice. The truth is that you can be trained to respond to a kind voice too. It is worth the risk to give yourself permission to pay less attention to the inner critic.

To Practice: Getting Curious about the Voices in Your Head

When the inner critic is the only or the loudest voice, we get caught in toxic inner narrative. To counter this tendency, let's identify some of the other voices that come and go during your day and get to know them:

- Your optimist: She's the one with the big ideas and the grand plans. What does she look and sound like?
- Your quirky one: You can count on her to start a sentence with "This might sound weird but . . ." Next time she shows up, reflect on the uniqueness she brings out.
- Your wise woman: Her voice often comes with a feeling of gravity. She's the one who has seen it all and responds with knowing.

What other voices would you add to this list and how do they show up? Identifying the diversity of voices in your internal landscape is powerful because it reminds you that, like with any story, there is more than one narrative. The critical voice might never completely disappear, but it can be balanced by all these other voices, which are much more productive.

ACKNOWLEDGE THAT PERFECTION DOES NOT EXIST

I recently had a patient, Sally, lament to me that she completely failed at real self-care. She had a work acquaintance who had been wanting to meet up on a weekend for months and months. This acquaintance was known to be toxic, but she wore Sally down with requests until Sally ended up saying yes and went to brunch with her one Sunday morning. When Sally got home from their brunch, she felt nearly sick. She was upset at herself for not holding her boundary, and she felt so clearly that she had not wanted to spend her precious free time on a person who brought nothing to her life. She reflected that in the past, she would have told herself, "I was being a good friend," but now she recognized, "This person isn't my friend, and I don't want her to be my friend."

Be careful here. There can be a strong tendency to beat yourself up when you aren't perfect with real self-care. And the thing is, you will never be perfect at real self-care. It's a constant process, not a destination. You do not need to be doing it perfectly right for it to work. In my session with Sally, we reframed the brunch incident as her *collecting data*: it was actually a win that after the meal she immediately recognized what was making her feel bad. That's what real self-care is—learning more about your true self, the part of you that has likes and dislikes, needs and preferences. It will take time to get it right, and that is perfectly normal. You'll make mistakes *even when* you're doing it right.

INVEST IN RECEIVING

Earlier this year, I was speaking to a woman who was going through a particularly difficult time in her life. Her kids had been dealing with some health issues, and we were still in the height of the pandemic. Life was a struggle. That said, this woman repeatedly emphasized how grateful and lucky she felt to have a full-time job and a supportive partner. "I know there are so many other people out there who have it a lot worse, so I should not be complaining." She went on to share about how her neighbor was a professional chef and one day offhandedly offered to cook her family a steak dinner and drop it off. She immediately and reflexively said no. Yes, it would have been wonderful and her mouth was literally watering as she said no, but she didn't deserve that type of handout. There were plenty of other people who needed it much more than she did.

One of the biggest factors that gets in the way of self-compassion is a stifled ability to receive help, because we feel we either do not deserve it or that we are not needy enough. Every day we are faced with news of people around the world who are faced with trauma, natural disaster, war, and famine. Who are we to accept help?

But what if instead of looking outward for permission to receive, we reframed accepting support, love, or attention from others as a skill that we need to build up? Esther Perel, a Belgian sex therapist, relationship expert, and author, commented, "In my culture, you ask a friend to babysit. Here, first you try to hire someone; then you go and 'impose.'"[6] I commonly see this play out in my practice. A patient of mine who is a mom of two found out her partner would be going on a last-minute work trip for two nights. Her sister, who lived in the same city, offered to come spend the night to help with the kids' bedtime and the morning routine. My patient's gut reaction was to dismiss the help: "It's only two nights, I'll be fine." I asked her why it was hard for her to say yes to a family member who was offering, and my patient said, "I don't want to inconvenience my sister; I know she has a lot on her plate as it is." Her automatic thought was to view herself as an imposition.

Yet, if we turn this situation upside down we can think about how it feels for the sister who is generously offering help to keep hearing no. Humans thrive on shared connection—instead of resisting and turning away supports in your life, remind yourself that the people who offer help are receiving as well.

To Practice: Microdosing Your Capacity to Receive

Just like setting boundaries, saying yes to offers of help or support can feel quite uncomfortable. Partly, this is because American culture exalts individualism and stoicism. We also dismiss and devalue the invisible labor that goes into caretaking work. As a result of this social conditioning, we just don't have enough practice receiving. So part of building up your self-compassion is finding small ways to say yes to help when it's offered. This practice also helps counter your tendency to move toward Martyr Mode. Try the following: The next time someone in your life offers a lending hand, pay attention to how quickly you jump to "No thanks . . . I'm okay!"

Even if the offer of help is not exactly what you had hoped for—for example, perhaps a friend offers to watch your kids on a Thursday after school, but you could use the help more on a Tuesday—practice saying yes anyway.

Letting yourself accept help is a critical skill that not only builds your support system in a tangible manner but also provides value for the help offerers. Each time you practice it, you're giving friends and family a chance to strengthen interpersonal bonds, which is beneficial for their well-being too.

GET CURIOUS ABOUT YOUR ANGER

Machik Labdrön, a female master and lineage holder of Buddhism, is reported to have remarked: "In other traditions demons are expelled externally. But in my tradition, demons are accepted with compassion."

Perhaps the most routinely loathed of any emotion is anger. If you find yourself working through these exercises and still having trouble softening your inner critic, there might be an underlying anger that has not been expressed. This could be anger at your life circumstances or specific people who are close to you, and in tandem, anger directed toward yourself. It's important to identify this anger because otherwise it will operate under the surface, covertly, while also coming out in destructive ways.

During the times in my life when self-compassion has been very difficult to access, I've first had to come to terms with my anger. For example, in the late 2000s, I was assigned a surgical rotation at a notoriously hostile hospital in Philadelphia. At the time, as a medical student, I was at the bottom of the ladder, waking up at 3:30 a.m. to make it into the hospital by 5:00 a.m. to pre-round on my assigned patients. If I was lucky, I was allowed to scrub in to the operating room to observe cases, where I once witnessed a senior surgeon angrily throwing equipment at staff during surgery. The dynamic between residents and attending surgeons was similar to what we experienced as students—one of disrespect and cruelty.

My response was to beat myself up internally for not studying enough, for not being the top student on rounds, and generally, in my opinion, for failing at life. I reached out to an adviser to try and make sense of what was going on. Through our conversation, though, I came to understand that I was angry. Not just angry—pissed! As a student I was there to learn, but instead of learning, I felt like I was being treated inhumanely—my team had never even bothered to learn my name. In those days, the words *toxic work environment* were not yet commonplace, and I'm not proud to admit I never reported any of this behavior (though there were folks above me who did). Interestingly, once I named my anger externally, my inner critic softened up. I had been taking the anger I had toward others out on myself.

I see this same phenomenon with my patients—women who have subtle or not-so-subtle anger lurking under the surface. Historically, our culture has not allowed women to feel their anger, and because of this, instead of turning toward their very real feelings of rage, my patients spend time asking if they are *allowed* to feel this way—if their feelings of anger are justified. The thing is, that's not how feelings work. Feelings are not rational actors. They just *are*. It's our job to learn how to feel them, and then we can decide if we want to take action based on them. Telling yourself that your anger isn't rational doesn't do anything to actually stop said anger; instead it creates more obstacles in the long run by obstructing your view of what's *really* going on.

CONNECT WITH YOUR BODY

On the topic of compassion, you have probably heard a lot of advice telling you to rest your body. The reason this advice is bountiful is because rest—including sleep, relaxation, time spent on activities that do not earn you money or status—is vitally important to our well-being.

However, what's missing from the conversation on rest is how to get yourself to do it when you're someone who is allergic to rest. You cannot rest your body unless you actually acknowledge that you *have* a body that needs rest. And you cannot acknowledge that your body is tired and needs rest unless you first develop some compassion for yourself. In other words, self-compassion is a prerequisite for embodiment, which in turn is a prerequisite for rest.

Disembodiment takes many forms—for example, mindlessly scrolling social media, forgetting to eat or drink water, exercising to the point of injury—but ultimately it leads to a lack of ability to make meaningful and productive choices for yourself. You might struggle with disembodiment if you can relate to these statements:

- When someone asks how you are feeling, it's impossible for you to name an emotion or a sensation in your body.
- You are blinded by a need for productivity or performance.
- You identify so strongly with Martyr Mode or shame-based thinking that it's difficult to connect with what you want or need in the moment.

A patient of mine, Naomi, recently made this connection for herself as she observed her elderly mother. Naomi's mother was in her seventies, with a long list of health ailments and chronic conditions. Yet she could not sit still. During an extended stay with Naomi, she was constantly bouncing from the kitchen to the garden to the grocery store and back again. And this was not an energetic or "happy to help!" type of existence—it was the type in which Naomi was constantly worried about whether her mother was going to fall and break her hip (again). The problem was that Naomi's mother was woefully disconnected from her body. She had spent a lifetime pushing herself to the max and was of a generation that eschewed admitting any sort of weakness or frailty.

Naomi's mother, quite predictably, overdid it and injured her wrist when working in the kitchen one day. But then her disembodiment went even further, as she was reluctant to seek medical care. What triggered Naomi in particular was that after her mother's injury, when she was finally forced to abstain from certain activities, her mother incessantly apologized for resting. Naomi developed a nonstop refrain of reminding her mother that she didn't need to say she was sorry for simply paying attention to the signals her body was sending her. This experience helped Naomi understand that she had the same underlying tendencies to push herself to the limit and to dismiss her body's cues for a break. Seeing her mother's patterns jolted Naomi into awareness and motivated her to start working on her own self-compassion.

Embodiment can look like being curious about ourselves, asking ourselves what our body needs in any given moment, and making the space to allow for that—whether it's rest, movement, or stimulation. Tricia Hersey is the founder of the Nap Ministry, a social justice movement based on the framework that rest is resistance against the systems of oppression we face in our daily lives. In an interview for *The New York Times*, Hersey said, "Being exhausted is not how we're supposed to be navigating this world. It's true trauma."[7] Through the Nap Ministry, Tricia educates women of color to empower themselves by choosing rest. It can be a nap or it can look like stepping away from your email or taking a walk around the block. It's less important what you do and more important that you understand that rest—as a type of self-compassion—is not a form of weakness but, instead, an assertion of strength.

If you're like me, rest, relaxation, and embodiment are tough choices to make. All the *doing* feels productive because it moves us forward. When we are still and resting, we must sit with the anxiety of being with ourselves and pay attention to our feelings and senses. For many, this stillness provokes anxiety. We want to quickly discharge the anxiety by doing something, *anything*. There can even be a sort of "high" that comes with checking off all the items on our lists.

Going a step further, when we look more closely at this pattern to forgo rest, what often comes to light is fear. There can be an underlying worry that if you were to finally put your feet up for a few minutes, if you were to say yes to support from others, if you were to be kind to yourself, you might just fall apart. When you finally do give yourself the space to connect with your body, it's likely that the first thing you will feel is how utterly exhausted you are. It can be easier to keep going, numb and empty, than to stop and feel fatigue when you rest.

Please, though, be brave. What would life feel like if we spent even just a little time being inside of and with ourselves? Self-compassion is a radical act of subversion of the social structures that are built to keep us quiet and overburdened. Envisioning acts of embodiment and rest as resistance can fill you with a sense of agency and control. Women have long practiced asserting this fierce self-compassion toward others—their families, their children, those whom they are responsible for. Now it's our job to take this stance toward ourselves. In the practice of real self-care, recognizing when you need rest and then employing boundaries and self-compassion to give yourself permission to take it, is critical. The more connected you feel to your body, the easier it is to make larger decisions from a place of clarity, which will be important for the next step of real self-care—identifying your values.

Of note, this is where practices like yoga, meditation, and mindfulness can be powerful tools to help you slow down and connect with your body. While yoga as faux self-care (e.g., performative or as avoidance of the work of real self-care) won't cut it, doing the work of real self-care to choose a body-based practice can be transformative.

To Practice: Choosing Rest

Rest is the place from which we derive physical and emotional energy, and energy is power. I think of rest as more of a stance than as any one particular action. So, when we decide to rest in whatever capacity that is, it's a single action that pushes against the social forces demanding our time, energy, and attention. Choosing rest is a revolutionary act. Your goal here is to start small and make microdecisions that are in favor of your body and your energy—as opposed to the people and entities that are asking for your attention.

The next time you find yourself overwhelmed, overworked, or just generally fried, take a minute to ask yourself the following questions:

1. What is my body trying to tell me right now?
2. What's one small thing I can do to take care of my body right now? (This might be as minuscule as allowing yourself to use the bathroom when you have the urge, versus holding it for several hours.)

3. What are the areas in my life where I can practice the skills of setting boundaries and softening my inner critic to allow me to choose rest?

The next time you find yourself overwhelmed, think about these steps you've just identified and put them into action. You'll find that even taking one small step in the service of rest goes a long way; each bit of rest that you take makes it easier to choose rest again.

SOUNDS GREAT, BUT . . .

Self-compassion is a tough nut to crack, so don't be alarmed if you have outstanding questions about how to put this work into practice. Here are some of the most common questions and critiques that come up on this topic.

Self-compassion sounds great and all, but what does any of this have to do with changing systems? Isn't real self-care supposed to be something that impacts the world at large and makes it a better place for everyone?

Let's revisit my patient Sonia, from earlier in the chapter, to get a better understanding of what self-compassion as revolution looks like in practice. After we identified Sonia's inner critic as the voice of her mother, Sonia made a some brave choices that stemmed from Good Enough: She decided to enroll her youngest child in daycare, and she asked for a long-promised increase in admin support at work. She also set boundaries with her mother, whose critical voice we had personified as Regina George from *Mean Girls*. Like with guilt, the voice did not go away, but she no longer consulted it or took Regina's critiques personally.

With the newfound permission that she felt, Sonia took a leap and started to tentatively embrace the idea of rest. She scheduled a babysitter to come one Sunday afternoon a month, and during that time, instead of catching up on her job, she rested her mind and body. She napped. She listened to her favorite true crime podcasts. She chatted with old friends and tried out new recipes.

Making this space for herself allowed Sonia to feel ready to process some of her anger, and it came out that she had felt unsupported by her partner, Brad, after she had their second child. Brad worked for a small start-up and, during the postpartum period with their second kid, had not taken paternity leave. Sonia never pushed him on this choice, but she had been carrying resentment around for almost two years at this point.

When she got pregnant with their third child a year later, she asked Brad to request paternity leave from his employer. Sonia understood that it was up to her to exert agency in her relationship, and that using her voice to express her needs was an assertion of power. Brad agreed and, though he was nervous about making a stir in such a small company, he went ahead and made the request. It turned out that he was the first male-identifying employee to ask for leave. The partners at his start-up decided that they wanted to provide good benefits to retain top talent, so they instituted a six-week paid paternity leave policy for all partners of birthing people in the office. This change would go on to impact all families in the workplace. And it started with Sonia learning how to treat herself with compassion.

As you can see, all four of the principles of real self-care must work in concert for a cascade effect to occur, and this work takes time. But as opposed to the momentary relief of getting a massage or signing up for a mindfulness class, this inner work is what propels change inside ourselves, and then in turn, in our families and the systems that we live and work in.

I struggle with self-compassion because my life is built on being a caretaker for several extended family members who, without me, would literally fall apart. On top of this, over the past few years, I've been through some devastating life circumstances (death of my partner), and I am also suffering from intergenerational trauma (my father was an alcoholic). But because of the sheer weight of the responsibilities on my shoulders, self-compassion always feels completely self-indulgent. The way I've pushed myself to be a caretaker for others is by being hard on myself—if I were to rest, others would suffer. In my mind, it's impossible for me to be nice to myself and also take care of others. I know this is not necessarily true or productive, but how do I change my thinking when every ounce of my body and mind fights against it?

What I hear in this question is someone who is dealing with a high level of emotional pain and is practiced at carrying the burden. When the level of suffering is high, I remind my patients that the next best step is to find a way to be curious about your pain. If you can muster it, even for five minutes, try holding your suffering with tenderness and asking what it wants to say to you.

We must always tailor real self-care to where we are on the map. And when you come from a family with intergenerational trauma, the work of speaking to yourself with respect and really believing that you do deserve rest and kindness can feel downright ludicrous because it was never positively modeled for you (in fact, it might have been viewed with suspicion or paranoia). Here, along with looking curiously at your suffering, try leaning into your anger. Where did you learn that you can only be useful to others if you don't feel your own feelings? Or did you learn that someone else will step in and save you? Working with a therapist, a psychiatrist, or a trusted adviser can be helpful when asking yourself these tough questions.

If you're the caretaker of elderly parents or young children, it's not uncommon to think about yourself as separate from the loved ones you are charged with supporting. Scott Stanley, PhD, a research professor and codirector of the Center for Marital and Family Studies at the University of Denver, suggests a framework of going from "Me to We" when working with couples, and I like applying this concept to caregiver situations. Your mental narrative might be: "I need to make sure that Dad makes it to all of his doctor appointments." Taking care of your own needs can easily get misconstrued as being in direct competition with the needs of others. Instead of getting caught in a competitive mindset (i.e., Me versus Them), reframe this to think of yourself as a team, wherein your needs and well-being are part of a larger system. This might look like: "What can I do to support myself so we make it to all of Dad's appointments?" You need to bring yourself into the picture and recognize that you are part of the We. Without your health and well-being, taking care of Them is impossible.

WHEN TO SEEK PROFESSIONAL HELP

I want to acknowledge that self-compassion as I described it here, while an important piece of real self-care, is not available for everyone all the time. If you are someone who has struggled with depression, anxiety, or other types of mental health problems in the past, you might find it particularly difficult to access self-compassion. When in the midst of a major depressive episode or a clinical anxiety episode, negative self-talk, like your inner critic, can become very, very loud—it's often the loudest voice in your head.

In Chapter 4, we discussed that self-care is not a treatment for clinical mental health conditions. As a reminder, instead of considering real self-care a cure, I like to think of it as a data point to keep track of how our interventions are going. For example, when I have a patient with a clinical mental health condition who can relatively easily access a feeling of Good Enough about herself, and who can set boundaries with her inner critic, we know that her depression or anxiety is being well managed. On the other hand, if someone who has previously been able to set boundaries with her inner critic is now plagued with negative self-talk, we know we need to adjust her treatment program.

Like with all the lessons we are learning in real self-care, remember, we cannot arrive at self-compassion using the same tools that drove us away from it. Perfectionism, self-criticism, and hyperfunctioning will not bring us to self-compassion. Ultimately, of the Four Principles of Real Self-Care, self-compassion is the one that requires the greatest permission for women. We have spent centuries in a culture that makes us invisible, demeans us, and tells us that we don't matter. Talking to yourself with kindness and respect, understanding that you are worthy of time and help, and realizing that you deserve rest are all radical acts. You are the only one who can give that permission to yourself. And for you, it might start off small, like catching a glimpse of self-compassion in the mirror—noticing your inner critic when it rears up or catching Marytr Mode soon after it occurs instead of letting it simmer for months.

The principles of real self-care build on each other and work synergistically. You can't be compassionate with yourself until you've learned to start saying no to others, and you also can't set boundaries unless you let go of some of your shame. Time and time again, you will find yourself working through one principle and quickly moving back to the one before. This is okay. Self-compassion for yourself and *for your own self-care practice* is vitally important.

THE SELF-COMPASSION CHECKLIST

Your quick reference when it comes to self-compassion

- Giving yourself *permission* leads to giving yourself *compassion*.
- Compassion is something you must give yourself; you can't expect it to always come from the outside.
- Your inner critic may have gotten you this far in life, but she is not the only voice that matters anymore.
- Perfectionism is an illusion that leads to loneliness, demoralization, and disconnection.
- You don't have to be down and out to accept help.
- Understanding your anger will help you get closer to self-compassion.
- Allowing yourself to rest is a strategy to reclaim your energy from toxic systems.
- Remember, what you are feeling is *betrayal*, not burnout.

Chapter 7

REAL SELF-CARE BRINGS
YOU CLOSER TO YOURSELF

BUILDING YOUR REAL SELF-CARE COMPASS

———

There's no such thing as balancing work and family. This language points us toward a problem to be solved, a destination at which we arrive. It is far more accurate to say that relationship with partner, relationship with children, and relationship with work exist as an ever-evolving, dynamic, and noisy conversation.

ALEXANDRA H. SOLOMON, PHD

My patient Rochelle, forty-five, is a white woman from California who had recently relocated to the East Coast. Rochelle had spent most of her life taking care of everyone around her. When her mother was sick, Rochelle moved in and coordinated all of her doctor appointments. When the family went through a financial crisis, Rochelle emptied her savings. In our work together, we identified that her role in the family was to be the savior. She was the one called when there was a problem that needed solving. And she was really, really good at it.

But after decades of this, Rochelle felt completely beholden to her parents and siblings and like there was no room for her. Through our work together, Rochelle learned that she had to set boundaries and start saying no to her family's demands. When her mother called her on a Saturday, insisting that she drop everything and come help fix her laptop, she demurred. When her sister asked her to fly back to California to help her find a new apartment, she passed. These were huge wins for Rochelle, and she was happy with herself for coming so far. But now she had a new problem—she had absolutely no idea what to do with herself when she wasn't catering to her family.

Rochelle's challenge was one I'd seen in many patients in my practice: once they've clearly identified what they don't want in their lives, they feel adrift, uncertain about what truly fills them up. Thankfully, once we've set our boundaries and begun to treat ourselves with more compassion, we have the mental space to reflect on what is truly nourishing and fulfilling to us.

It all begins with identifying our values.

This chapter will teach you the third principle of real self-care, which is that real self-care brings you closer to yourself. It looks different for everyone, but it means that you feel connected with your values and are engaged in activities that align with them. Identifying our values in an explicit way emboldens us to make clear choices. And those choices lead to purpose and a sense of fulfillment.

GOALS VERSUS VALUES: WHO YOU ARE WHEN YOU'RE TRAVELING IS WHO YOU ARE WHEN YOU GET THERE

To begin, let's clarify the difference between goals and values, because they're easy to confuse. Goals are tangible objectives like "I want to run a marathon," or "I want to get into graduate school." Values, on the other hand, are desired qualities of action. You can embody your values while you are working toward your goals (and even if you fail at your goals). So, if I'm training to run a marathon, what value do I embody while I'm training? Is it a sense of adventure in trying something new? Or is it a sense of courage in the face of a difficult challenge?

Put another way, if goals are the things that you do, values are the way that you do them. Imagine your life as one long road trip. Your goals would include each destination you arrive at, whether you're pulling in to the Grand Canyon or taking a break at a roadside pit stop. Your values are how it feels for you to be in the car, driving toward the various destinations on this trip. Are you singing along to your favorite '80s hip-hop? Are you engrossed in a rousing game of I spy with your kids? Or are you white-knuckled and cursing traffic? The distinction is important because the way you move toward your goals influences the mental and physical state you're in when you arrive.

You may have noticed that the faux self-care coping strategies from Chapter 2 are all aligned with concrete goals, as opposed to values. We go on a wellness retreat with the goal of escaping our daily lives; we do a juice cleanse to lose weight. And typically, we believe that we will feel better once we achieve our goals. Rarely do we identify the values underneath them. Rather, we use faux self-care as a goal-oriented coping strategy to deal with overwhelm and disconnection from our values. The work of real self-care is deeper; it's a process to help you live by your values. Remember, real self-care is not a thing to do—it's a way to be.

But here's the kicker. If you're anything like me or my patients, it's easy for you to put blinders on and get hyperfocused on goals. Give me a checklist and I am off to the races. The problem with this way of living is that you end up missing out on what matters most in life. Values are not only descriptors of *how* you want to live your life but also *why* you make the decisions that you do. No two people have the same constellation of values.

As we touched on in Chapter 4, research tells us that people who develop authentic meaningful relationships and who are in touch with their purpose in life are happier and more fulfilled. When you have tunnel vision for your goals and forget about why those goals matter to you, you run the risk of feeling empty inside and dipping into burnout or worse—depression or anxiety.

In his work on acceptance and commitment therapy, Dr. Russ Harris defines values as "our heart's deepest desires for the way we want to interact with the world, other people, and ourselves."[1] Our values, then, are about how we want to show up.

What sort of person do you want to be? What *really* matters to you? Taking committed action in line with your values is nourishing because it brings you closer to yourself and, in the process, promotes eudaimonic well-being. In short, being connected with your values helps you *feel*, and being able to feel your feelings is critical in the practice of real self-care.

This chapter is divided into two sections: The first will illustrate tools and exercises that will help you get in the mindset of thinking about your values and you will create your Values List. In the second section, we will use your Values List to build your Real Self-Care Compass.

As you work your way through these tools, remember the importance of setting boundaries and embracing self-compassionate narratives. Real self-care is an iterative process that requires you to hold all of these principles in mind and, with practice, becomes second nature.

BUILDING YOUR VALUES LIST

Here's a short list of common values to reference as you read through the chapter. Please note this list is not meant to be exhaustive, but to jump-start your process of identifying your own. Read through this list and underline the values that resonate most with you (without stopping to second-guess yourself). Then, as you work through the "To Practice" tools over the next few pages, add more values as they come up in your answers.

ACCEPTANCE	KINDNESS	HOPE
AUTONOMY	RESPONSIBILITY	LEADERSHIP
ADVENTURE	INTEGRITY	COMPASSION
CARING	TRUSTWORTHINESS	COMMUNITY
AUTHENTICITY	SELF-AWARENESS	PLAYFULNESS
BELONGING	HUMILITY	BOLDNESS
FREEDOM	HONESTY	LEARNING
CREATIVITY	COURAGE	OPENNESS
CURIOSITY	FLEXIBILITY	STABILITY
UNDERSTANDING	RISK TAKING	SERVICE
GENEROSITY	HUMOR	SPIRITUALITY
JUSTICE	STEADFASTNESS	

You may be wondering, "How do I even identify my values, much less make decisions in line with them?" In the following pages, I'll guide you through this process by introducing a set of tools to help you grasp which activities, interests, and qualities nourish your true sense of self.

CHOOSE ONE VALUE OVER ANOTHER

Values are most easy to discern when we consider them in the context of decisions. Bethany Saltman is a coach and author who helps individuals and teams run their businesses aligned with their values. In founding my women's mental health company, Gemma, my team and I worked with Bethany to get clarity in making big decisions that we were facing about the direction of the company. Bethany emphasizes that a value is most useful when it is framed as choosing one quality over another. So, for example, in the business world, defining your company's values could mean choosing justice *over* stability or prioritizing customer service *over* flexibility. For Gemma, this meant getting clarity that our relationships as friends and colleagues were more important than the speed at which we got our next product into the market. This broader values framework can also be applied to individuals.

Take, for example, my patient Kleo. Kleo and her wife, Melanie, had recently saved up enough money to buy their dream home and were renovating the kitchen. Melanie lamented that Kleo had everything she said she had wanted (and that she'd worked so hard to achieve), yet she seemed miserable about all of it. I noticed this too—in our sessions together, Kleo often rattled off laundry lists of to-dos and projects, and seemed to feel burdened or oppressed by them.

Kleo and I spent time reflecting on what was going on and looking at how she could make some clear choices that were in line with her values. For example, in most areas of her life, Kleo valued making bold decisions—she was one of the first women to rise in the ranks at her company, and coming out as a teenager had clarified for her that acting in accordance with what was true for her was of the utmost priority. She was happier when she was embracing the unique parts of herself than when she turned the volume down to fit in.

In renovating her new home, however, Kleo found herself dead inside as she scrolled sites like Pinterest, looking for inspiration. She felt limited by the rules of how a "dream home" was supposed to look. It seemed this kitchen remodel was bringing up some old baggage for Kleo. She had grown up poor in a cramped apartment with five siblings. Her parents never had the resources to buy new furniture, let alone remodel a house. Kleo had worked her butt off to get to where she was financially, and to some extent, the kitchen remodel was an "I've made it" of sorts. But she noticed that there was a hidden script running in her mind, pushing her toward an upper-middle-class design aesthetic. It screamed beige, and Kleo felt suffocated.

Once we discovered what was going on, we came up with a plan for Kleo to set aside dedicated time to allow her imagination to run wild. She went to the bookstore and let herself browse the magazine aisle, picking out home décor colors and themes that brought her joy. In the end, Kleo picked out a bright blue kitchen island and patterned tiles that reminded her of her honeymoon in Puerto Rico. Allowing herself to show up as authentically herself, even if it wasn't "on trend," lit Kleo up inside and reminded her that this project was her own. Yes, it was true that if her family ever decided to sell this home, they'd have a tough sell with the design of the kitchen. However, making this clear choice— boldness and authenticity over prudence and self-restraint—was aligned with her values. While her wife wasn't as gung ho about a blue kitchen as Kleo, Melanie was thrilled to see the spark back in Kleo's eyes and happy to be along for the ride.

The clarity that comes from making a clear decision and from understanding *why* you are making this decision is energizing. When you make a proactive choice, instead of feeling like your life is being done to you, you're practicing real self-care.

Systemic constraints are always at play in the foreground or background (more so if you come from a marginalized group). So, the ability to make a clear choice about what we do with our time is a privilege in itself. Again, that's why real self-care has the potential to be such a transformative act; we are making an internal shift within ourselves to reject the toxic cultural messaging we have ingested for far too long.

When you do the work of choosing one value over another, like Kleo did in renovating her kitchen, your brain will understandably have the tendency to overvalue certain words (service, connection, love) and undervalue others (ambition, freedom, playfulness). Yet, remember that the work of identifying your values is clearly grounded in the fact that all of us are *different* and that our difference is our power. Kleo, for example, got understandably caught up in what she was "supposed" to want. Overly identifying with the "shoulds" in our lives—whether that's in regard to a kitchen remodel or to a bigger decision like career choice or whether or not to have children—always takes us away from our values. When I'm working with patients, I can usually see a clear line going from the statement "well, I should want . . ." to "everyone else is doing. . . ." It's human nature to want to fit in with your family, community, or culture, and if everyone else around you is picking out a beige kitchen island, it's understandable that you'd sometimes forget that you don't even like the color. Clearly articulating our values for ourselves helps us counteract the "shoulds" and the comparisons.

If you're feeling tempted to beat yourself up about your tendency to want to fit in with the pack, please don't. This instinct is hardwired into us, and it takes awareness and practice to undo it. For example, researchers from Johns Hopkins University found that children as young as two years old will change their decision-making based on social influence by their peers.[2] This study highlights how even at such a young age, children understand that it's socially advantageous to stick with the crowd. While this adaptive defense mechanism certainly helped from an evolutionary standpoint, it doesn't serve us the same way now, wherein what makes us unique is important to our own well-being.

To Practice: Your Birthday Dinner

You're throwing a birthday dinner party for yourself, and have a budget of two hundred dollars. Think about what the party looks like and how you come to your decisions about the event. With a constrained budget, what choices do you make? Things to consider: How many people will you invite? Will you make it a potluck? Where will the party happen? Will there be a theme? Be careful here not to get caught up in the "shoulds"—this is an imaginary dinner party, and the point of this exercise is to let your brain imagine how you'd dream this up, without judgment. Now answer the following questions:

1. Imagine the scene of the party itself. Write down the three to five values that stand out to you immediately, and that describe how you went about your decision-making. Reference the values list at the beginning of the chapter if you need help. Remember, there are no right answers here. Just what's true for you.

2. When faced with the presentation of the event (where it's held, who is invited, what food is served) versus how you and the guests feel when they are at your dinner, which is more important to you? How do you weigh these items?

This exercise not only provides you with values that you can add to your Values List, it's also a reminder that no two of us will make the same choices for our dinner party. There is no one "right way" to celebrate your birthday, in the same way there is no one "right way" to live your life.

MATCH YOUR INSIDES AND YOUR OUTSIDES

A couple of years ago my patient Jolene came to me distraught. She was in her midtwenties, and all of her friends were getting engaged and seemingly riding off into the sunset with their supposed White Knights. Meanwhile, Jolene was woefully single and had never had a serious relationship.

"Dr. Lakshmin," she said, "there's no hope for me. I'm doomed to be alone forever."

With a good deal of compassion, I said, "What makes you believe that when you find 'the One' you'll be riding off into the sunset, living an easy breezy life of happily ever after?"

This was a question Jolene had never once considered. She equated reaching her goal—of finding a partner and starting a family—with blissful happiness. She didn't stop to think about *who* she was outside of these milestones or the fact that achieving these goals was not in itself guaranteed to bring her inner bliss.

In our work together, we spent time redirecting Jolene from feeling bad about her single life to practicing what made her fulfilled. She began to understand that she would not suddenly change or become "fixed" just because she found a boyfriend or a husband. In fact, the more difficult work of learning how to be in an adult partnership would start once she found a relationship.

Many of us spend our time thinking, "Once I land that pro-motion, then I'll be a new and better version of myself," or "Once I have X amount of money saved, my life will be a little bit easier, then I'll be happy." And, on one hand, economic security and relational stability are both real endeavors that do provide sys-temic advantages. But they are not cure-alls for what an adviser of mine called "the problems of living."

Interestingly, as Jolene started to explore her own interests and passions, she came to realize that she had been looking in all the wrong places for a partner. She was getting set up with straitlaced, Wall Street–type guys at the behest of friends and family members. But on the inside, Jolene was a free-spirited, goofy person. She didn't take herself too seriously. She loved making people laugh. So she started going to comedy meetup shows around the city and getting to know folks who moved in creative circles. Jolene ended up dating a man who made guitars for a living and, on the side, was an aspiring comic. When she was with him, she felt like she could be herself. The outsides of her life looked a bit different than what she imagined they would be—marrying a man who didn't have the career stability or the income potential of many of her friends and colleagues meant a much more modest wedding and a honeymoon spent camping. But on the other hand, Jolene felt joyful and fulfilled with her partner, as opposed to just checking off boxes.

It's a risk to live life by your values because your decisions might put you at odds with those closest to you, or you might find yourself "falling behind" in culturally held metrics like money, status, or prestige (or, conversely, self-sacrifice and devotion to caretaking). The thing is, not only will culture (the expectations put on us from the outside) and your nature (your innate wants, needs, desires, preferences) sometimes clash, but perhaps even more important to understand is that the culture often gives women contradictory goals that are impossible to meet simultaneously. You're supposed to cook a photo-worthy meal every night while caring for your aging parents, but also climb to the top of the corporate ladder and have the money to buy a vacation home—What? When? How?

In her book *The Way of Integrity*, Martha Beck writes about her own experiences failing to recognize these contradictions.[3] Regarding a point of overwhelm and deep self-criticism in her life, Beck writes, "I was intensely confused. I didn't realize that I had picked up two sets of cultural beliefs that contradicted each other. My error of innocence lay in not seeing this contradiction and trying to fulfill both sides of two mutually exclusive codes for living."

The antidote to mutually exclusive codes for living? Turn inward instead of looking outward. Use values to more clearly understand what you want and need to live a full life.

Values work involves making sure your outsides match your insides. So Lucy, who loves art and thrives when she has access to open spaces, would be miserable in her job as a corporate attorney (spoiler alert: she was), and Becca, who craves structure and loves the feeling of accomplishment, would melt into a puddle if she spent her free time in a band. There are pros and cons to all of these choices—but when you make a life decision that aligns with your values, with your *insides*, then you don't care about what you're missing out on. It's only when your life is out of alignment with your values that you end up conflicted, miserable, and unable to stop yourself from binge-watching five episodes of *Law & Order: Special Victims Unit*. (Though, to be fair, I've been there, and nothing beats watching Mariska Hargitay catch the bad guy!)

WHEN TO SEEK PROFESSIONAL HELP

If you find yourself having a hard time connecting to what's on the inside—your feelings and your private thoughts—you might be engaging in numbing behaviors. Traditionally, when someone feels chronically numb, clinicians wonder about untreated trauma, and addiction and overuse of substances like alcohol as well. It's also important to consider addiction that does not meet the level of a clinical disorder but still prevents you from connecting to your values. This could take the form of turning to alcohol or drugs when your feelings get too intense, or using other distraction techniques like shopping, gambling, workaholism, food, sex, or even repeatedly engaging in conflict-filled relationships. If you are worried about a feeling of numbness that you can't shake, it's best to seek an evaluation with a mental health professional.

RUN TOWARD TOUGH DECISIONS

About six years ago I was faced with a tough professional decision. In my work as a physician at George Washington University, I had been building an academic career in global mental health. I had the opportunity to design a small research project in my extended family's home of Bangalore, India, studying women with depression and anxiety. Another meaningful project involved testimonial therapy to help immigrant survivors of intimate partner violence. I was working on this grand vision of bridging the world my family came from and researching therapeutic interventions that could impact women everywhere.

Simultaneously, freed by the work I'd done with my own therapist and healing from my time in the cult, I'd starting writing for small websites and blogs about the tyranny of self-care, the problematic nature of wellness, and the constraints women faced in the world. I started an Instagram account where I shared some of my own personal struggles and provided mental health education to my audience of mostly American women. My ideas were resonating with a wide audience and I found fulfillment in speaking to women who shared similar life experiences to me and my patients.

I felt like I was being pulled in two distinct directions—both of which were attractive to me, and both of which I had the professional credentials to excel in. But the reality was that it would be very difficult for me to become a grant-funded, academic, global mental-health researcher *and* to focus on writing that was more geared to the general public.

During this time in my life, I spent a good deal of energy getting clear on my values. Like most people, I admittedly love praise and being told I'm doing a great job. But, personality-wise, when I looked closely at my values, what rose to the surface was creativity and connection. I put my decision off for a couple of years, and during that time, I watched myself burn out from trying to simultaneously pursue two career paths. Interestingly, the burnout served as a clarifying force, in that writing for a general audience came much easier to me than the research work. I felt energized by the email responses I received when women read my work. Connecting with an audience similar to my patients (and to me) on social media was something I enjoyed and that came naturally. While I liked the research involved in global health because I was curious by nature, when I considered the politics of academia and the prospect of endless grant applications, I wanted to run for the hills. Moreover, I was noticing that while women in low- and middle-income countries struggle with a different set of stressors, there was some overlap in what I was seeing in that research and in the women I treated in Washington, DC. Granted, a career as an author or an entrepreneur was not going to be a walk in the park, either—but being my own boss suited me in a way that a career as an academic researcher was never going to. I was fortunate: as a physician, I was in a position to take a pay cut to pursue the path I chose, and I had a partner with health insurance benefits, which allowed me to stay in therapy.

A couple of years into this journey, I began writing for *The*

New York Times and had the chance to interview one of the foremost researchers in my field. I was shaking with nerves when I got on the phone with her, and I'm sure I said something completely uncool as we started our conversation. I was shocked when she said to me, "Pooja, thank you so much for what you're doing for our field. Your writing is bringing attention to women's mental health in a way that is so needed." Here was the expert of experts in my field, who represented the pinnacle of the path not traveled, telling me that my unique path was *also* valuable. Whereas I had always been trained to put certain life paths up on a pedestal—research, academic medicine—she reminded me that good things happen when all of us embrace our unique values and strengths, as opposed to trying to just steer ourselves into the same cookie-cutter mentality.

I imagine you can think back on times in your life when there was a fork in the road and you had to prioritize what really mattered to you. Maybe it was in high school, having to decide whether to pursue sports or music, or maybe it was as an adult making a choice between becoming a stay-at-home parent and remaining in the paid workforce.

Keep in mind these two truths:

- When you are at a fork in the road, you must pick a path. If you try to pursue too much at the same time, you will burn out and neither road will fulfill you.
- Your guide in making these tough decisions must be internal— your values—not external.

To Practice: What I Know to Be True for Me

Answer these questions with the first thought that comes to mind (no editing!) and save it into the notes app on your phone.

Quick trick: If you find it impossible to fill out this list yourself, you can enlist a proxy to answer the questions—someone who knows you very well and is capable of being in service to your goal of practicing real self-care. In other words, don't pick your overly critical work friend.

1. I'm happiest when _____.
2. I feel most like myself when I am _____.
3. I am bound to fail when _____.
4. I know that I cannot do ____ and be ____.

Now read through your sentences and see what values match up with your responses. Some of them might be contradictory, and that's okay. People are complicated, and two seemingly opposing things can both be true. When faced with a tough decision, come back to this list as a reminder of what you know to be true for you.

THE RELATIONSHIP BETWEEN ANXIETY AND LIVING BY YOUR VALUES

If you dial back from being goal oriented and embrace your values, will you be less productive and accomplish less? The true but scary answer is *yes*—you will be less productive *and* that's a good thing. If you are someone who has spent your life being goal oriented or performance minded, there's a good chance that you've been living with a bit of healthy anxiety. Anxiety isn't a bad thing—it's what gets us out of bed on time and forces us to meet deadlines. However, a key differentiator between people who practice real self-care and those who do not is developing the ability to prioritize and make a meaningful choice about how they spend their time. When your anxiety is in the driver's seat, everything feels very important and facing fork-in-the-road decisions can feel like failure.

Somewhat paradoxically, when you start shifting your decision-making to align with your values, you might become less productive and no longer able to meet the needs of those around you with the same timeliness or concern. This can cause *more* anxiety for you in the beginning. Yet, in the long run, you'll be doing fewer of the things that matter most to other people (or to society) and more of the things that matter most to you.

DIGEST WHAT'S IN FRONT OF YOU

When you're too goal-focused, you spend too much time in the problem-solving part of your brain, and you miss out on the good feelings that come when you achieve your goals. In other words, you can be at risk for becoming desensitized or numb to the good stuff in your life. So, it follows that part of removing addiction to goals and connecting with values is to *feel and internalize* your accomplishments. The practice of gratitude helps with this process. I think of gratitude not as counting your blessings but as a form of digestion, an idea derived from Buddhist teachings.

Jack Kornfield, a Western Buddhist master and author, has said, "We can either be lost in a smaller state of consciousness—what in Buddhist psychology is called the 'body of fear,' which brings suffering to us and to others—or we can bring the quality of love and appreciation, which I would call gratitude, to life. With it comes a kind of trust."[4] When we pay attention to the fruits of what we have in our life already, whether that is the small pleasures like our morning cup of coffee or bigger achievements like a job promotion or a healthy family—we actively engage with what is real and true in our world. And the reality is that for all of us, there is good along with the bad—no matter how burned out or drained we feel in the moment. The purpose of gratitude in this context doesn't involve toxic positivity or self-delusion. Rather, gratitude is a practice to tune your attention to what you have, so that you can then go on to appreciate what future good stuff will come your way. When you're lacking this skill, you'll forever be focused on the bad stuff, and even when the next gift arrives at your front door, you'll be worried that it's in the wrong wrapping paper.

We all have a certain level at which we can't absorb any more good stuff. When good things are happening in your life, there's a way that you can become numb to them. You work your ass off to buy your dream home. And after living in it for a few months, it's routine. You're ready for bigger and better. Why does this happen? Partly because we become habituated. But also, we don't spend enough time *digesting* the good stuff on a regular basis. We buy into the illusion that the next thing around the corner is going to fix all our problems or take away our insecurities. When you don't digest, you get full and bloated and cranky. You can't take any more in. You'll just keep collecting more experiences or things but won't ever feel nourished by them.

A patient of mine who was in the throes of the sandwich generation (i.e., caretaking her teenage kids while also tending to her ailing parents) experienced what it felt like to take notice of the good in her life and appreciate it. She had been feeling increasingly bogged down by the constant stream of activities, doctor appointments, and obligations that were required of her, and had very little connection to any good feelings related to her family. Then, one evening, her parents and kids were all around the kitchen table, playing a board game, teasing each other, just having a grand time. In our session, my patient reflected to me how fulfilling it was to watch this deep connection between the generations in her family, and to know that the time she put in shuffling everyone around made this bond possible. She internalized the good and felt satisfied.

Only when you fully acknowledge the wealth you have in life

can you be ready for more. And a funny thing happens when you start appreciating and digesting all the good: You stop caring as much about getting that next thing. You realize that what you have right now is just as good as what you may have in the future.

To Practice: Letting Yourself Have the Good Stuff

It can be difficult to recognize the good stuff in the moment and digest it in real time. It's easier to pick out memories from the past—hindsight gives us twenty-twenty vision. In this practice, you'll build your digestion skills by reflecting on past good stuff and the accompanying values—then you'll connect them to what's good in your life right now.

1. Name a few peak experiences or top moments from your life over the past few years. Try to identify a mix of big things, like finding your partner or starting your dream job, and also more subtle moments, like that time you read your favorite book all in one sitting, curled up on your front porch.

2. Now, with the vision and perspective you have today, imagine you are having a conversation with yourself as you were living through the peak moments. What do you wish you had known? What do you want yourself to hold on to about the magic moments in your life? What wisdom would you like to impart to that version of yourself about what was most important about these peaks?

3. Take it a step further and apply the language of values: Is there a value that you were living at that time that you would name now? What was *most* important to you in those moments that you could not see then, but that you can see very clearly now? Can you identify an associated value?

We all have these peak experiences, yet we so rarely sit down and reflect on why they felt good. By taking the time to explicitly name our values, we can use them to inform future decisions so that we are setting ourselves up for more experiences that are truly nourishing.

CHANNEL FLEXIBILITY WHEN YOUR VALUES SHIFT

When I was in my early thirties, after coming out the other side of a divorce, I was convinced that another marriage and children were not for me. On our second date, I told my now partner, Justin, that I wanted to live a vagabond life, and that I would never ever *ever* have kids. He was down with that, and we lived a life of freedom and independence into our late thirties.

Now, years later, here we are owning a home in Austin, and starting a family. In my early thirties, the values that were highest priority for me were independence and freedom. I needed to have the space to truly explore myself—my sexuality, my creativity, my understanding of the world. I grew up in a culture that did not make room for girls or women to do this, and so I found a way (albeit somewhat destructively at first). Over time, however, these priorities changed.

Our values are always shifting and seesawing. It's not a contradiction—it's human nature. It's helpful to remember that in each season of your life, you will have different priorities. This does not discount any one set of values; it's only a sign of change and growth.

Even now, as I'm on the precipice of having a baby, I'm up against another transition and values shift. Due to my past experiences, while my friends were building their families, I spent most of my thirties ambivalent about motherhood and unable to imagine myself in the role. I also did not want to rush my relationship with Justin. As a result, one reason I've been able to achieve the professional success that I have up until this point is because in those critical years my time was singularly my own. I'm terrified that when I become a mother, I'll lose what I have built. This fear is understandable and normal—every time our values shift, we may find ourselves feeling insecure or uncertain.

As any of us transition into a new season of life, we can carry some values forward with us, though they may manifest in unique ways. For example, my patient who is a graphic designer deeply values creativity and working with others. She embodies both of those values when she is with her team at their design firm, *and* she embodies it on Sunday afternoons when she works in the garden with her partner, plotting together which plants to try and where to place them, and designing a backyard that feels calming for them. Naming and recognizing the continuity in her values provided a sense of stability.

These times of transition are fruitful periods when it comes to identifying our values. When you're in between "here" and "there" you have the unique opportunity to imagine what's next and make your values even more explicit, and in this way, you are claiming ownership of your decisions.

Now that you have completed the "To Practice" sections of this chapter, take stock of your Values List and add additional values that come to mind. Keep your Values List handy as you read on for the next step in the real self-care practice—building your Compass.

YOUR REAL SELF-CARE COMPASS

You've probably heard of the concept of following your North Star. Leaders often talk about their North Star as a personal vision statement—a motto of sorts that helps you make decisions as you move through life. Yet, as we know, it's common for our values to shift as we move through transitions in life. Some will stay the same and new ones will pop up. Therefore, instead of looking for a North Star, when it comes to real self-care, I want you to build a *Compass*. A Compass makes room for shifting values and priorities and will be your guide in practicing real self-care.

To work through the next section of the chapter, you will need to set aside at least an hour of time when you can be by yourself. Try to clear your mind and find a space where you can concentrate. The internal work of connecting with your values and making decisions based on them may not always feel easy. If you're having one of those days when you need to flop on the couch and just watch Netflix, that's okay. Rest when you need it and come back to building your Compass when you have the energy to tackle it.

The Real Self-Care Compass is built on three questions: **WHAT**, **HOW**, and **WHY**.

We start by identifying your **WHAT**. Pick one goal for each specific area of your life—for your career or education, for your family life, and just for you. These are your **WHAT**s.

Next, with your Values List from earlier in the chapter in front of you, reflect deeply on **HOW** you want to accomplish these goals. Remember the birthday party exercise: there are many different ways to achieve your goals, and the key here is to get clear on how *you* want to achieve them—not how your boss wants you to achieve them or how your parents want you to achieve them.

After you've gotten clear on your **HOW**, think about your **WHY**. Your **WHY** is your personal manifesto and speaks to the raw truth of what feeds and nourishes you, and only you.

To give you an idea of what this looks like, here's my version, which I used when I started writing this book and when I began my IVF journey:

WHAT: *(My goal)* Write a book about how we've got self-care all wrong, and what we need to be doing instead.

HOW: *(My values)* With boldness, with authenticity, with compassion for myself and my readers

WHY: *(My personal manifesto)* Because what feeds me is connection, meaningful conversation, and understanding the internal world of myself and others.

WHAT: Expand my family

HOW: With compassion for myself, with flexibility, with trust

WHY: Because what feeds me is taking the risk to experience new roles, discovering more about myself, and deepening my relationship with Justin.

WHAT: Learn to rollerblade

HOW: With excitement, with an open mind, with curiosity

WHY: Because what feeds me is exploration, novelty, and teaching myself to do new things.

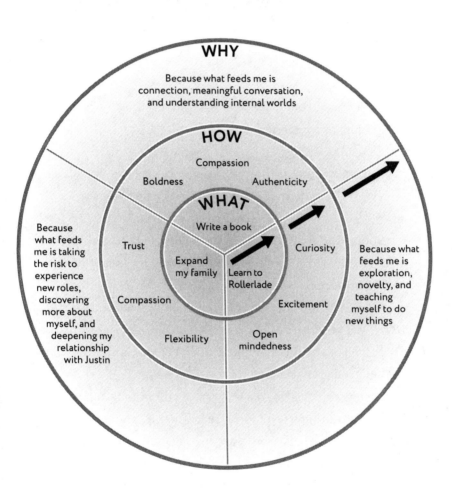

POOJA'S REAL SELF-CARE COMPASS

WHY
Because what feeds me is connection, meaningful conversation, and understanding internal worlds

HOW
Compassion
Boldness
Authenticity

WHAT
Write a book
Trust
Expand my family
Learn to Rollerlade
Curiosity
Compassion
Excitement
Flexibility
Open mindedness

Because what feeds me is taking the risk to experience new roles, discovering more about myself, and deepening my relationship with Justin

Because what feeds me is exploration, novelty, and teaching myself to do new things

Now it's your turn.

Pick one goal for each area of your life listed below.

- Family Life (parents, kids, partners, friendships)
- Career or Education
- Just for You

After that, fill out **HOW**s and **WHY**s for each, using the following prompt as a reference:

- **HOW**: *Your values (with compassion, with boldness, with ___)*
- **WHY**: *Your personal manifesto (because what feeds me is ___)*

Notice that your **WHAT**s can be big life goals (e.g., my goal to have a baby) or relatively small goals (e.g., my fascination with getting into rollerblading).

Now, using the blank Compass on page 195, transfer the **WHAT**, **HOW**, and **WHY** that you've compiled above onto the Compass. Your Compass is a visual representation of your goals, your values, and your personal manifestos, all combined.

You'll notice that goals are in the center of the Compass, as opposed to the outer layer, because in real self-care, as you know, our goals are secondary. Instead, our values are what guide us.

So, for example, when I started writing this book, I felt the inspiration to learn how to rollerblade. I had just moved to Austin and wanted a new hobby that got me outside and active. I regret to tell you that the pair of Rollerblades I bought about six months ago are still in the back of my closet. But I took the values and the personal manifesto from the rollerblading goal, and I brought them both to my life in the year I was writing this book and trying to expand our family. I tried not to be rigid with the process of writing and editing (*open-mindedness*), and I allowed myself to ask questions as to how real self-care was showing up in my patients and in myself as I went through IVF (*curiosity*). I repeatedly reminded myself that doing new things—like writing a book for the first time—is hard, *and* it's always been something that feeds me (*exploration and novelty*). In this way, you can practice real self-care even as you are working toward your goals.

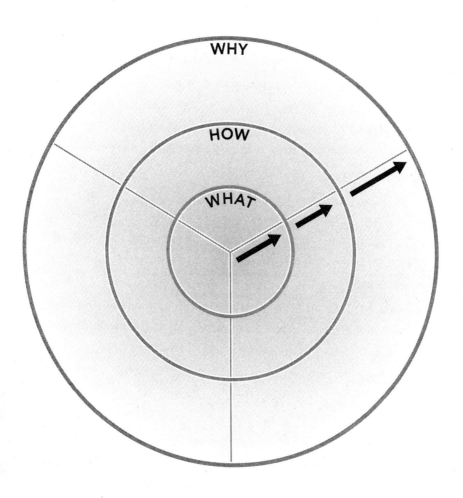

Use your Real Self-Care Compass to help guide day-to-day decisions about how to spend your time and energy, *and* when you are contemplating bigger life decisions. When faced with a tough request from a friend or family member, turn to your Compass to remind you of where your priorities lie. When planning a trip or considering a vacation, use your Compass to guide what type of trip you go on, and how (or if) you spend time with family. You can also consult your Compass when you are contemplating more weighty life decisions like switching jobs or moving. Keep versions of it in easily accessible places (e.g., your phone's home screen or a printout on your fridge or bathroom mirror). You want to feel grounded in this vision.

When you accomplish a goal, you can either add another one that aligns with those values and your personal manifesto *or* you can rework your manifesto to make a completely new direction in the Compass.

For extra credit, you can expand this list to include more life areas—for example, physical or spiritual health—or separate out nonfamily relationships and friendships.

STAYING ON COURSE

Now that you have your Compass and you're using it to guide your decision-making, it's natural to wonder if it's leading you in the right direction when it comes to your real self-care practice. To stay on the course of real self-care, you'll need to keep practicing the other principles too. Keep an eye out for the three yellow flags (see page 76). Occasionally take stock of where you are by returning to the Real Self-Care Thermometer on page 86.

And remember: Real self-care is not a religion, nor is your Compass. I am providing some guideposts and structures here *and* I encourage you to adapt these tools to work for you. Real self-care is not a thing to *do*—it's a way to *be*.

To see this in practice, let's go back to my patient Rochelle, who learned to set boundaries with her family, but then had no idea what she wanted to do with her newfound time. In our work together, we identified a value that was consistent across multiple aspects of Rochelle's life—self-expression. We brainstormed together how to bring forward the value of self-expression in her life. She remembered that as a girl, she used to journal. As she got older and life got busy, she stopped making time for writing. So, in service of real self-care, Rochelle blocked out an hour a week to write. Initially, the writing took the form of journaling, and was just for her. Over time, she decided to submit short essays to blogs and websites. This was not paid work, but instead a hobby that fed and nourished Rochelle and was aligned with one of her core values. In parallel, in her workplace, she started advocating for herself more and asked for a raise at her yearly review—again, embodying the value of self-expression and speaking up for what mattered to her. Through explicitly identifying her values, Rochelle understood that she had choices about how she spent her time and energy.

This feeling of ownership over your life is the goal of real self-care—and once you have it, you'll never want to lose it again.

SOUNDS GREAT, BUT . . .

What do I do when it feels like it's impossible to make choices based on my values because everyone else in my life will be disappointed, or even angry, with me?

When it comes to values and practicing real self-care, 99 percent of the questions that I get tie back (once again!) to how to handle disappointing people in your life. This is why learning to set boundaries and deal with guilt is the first principle of real self-care.

We live in a system that has never presented women with a full option of choices. Our social structures have constructed an environment where women's unpaid labor is the default. So, by definition, when you start pulling back from happily acquiescing to everyone around you and start making decisions based on your own values, people are going to have some feelings. If anything, anger from people who have taken you for granted or expected you to martyr yourself for them is a sign that you are on the right path. When you find yourself getting hung up on the feeling that using your Compass is impossible or that it would disappoint too many people, that's a sign to turn back to Chapter 5 of this book, and recommit to your practice of saying no. It's also a time to brush up on self-compassion (see Chapter 6), as it might be the case that your inner critic is preventing you from making choices aligned with your Compass.

Here, I also like to remember the tenet of We. For people who are truly on your team (your children, partner, closest friends), you being more full of life and mentally well is better for them. Those who cannot see your well-being as a positive in their own lives are not part of your We. This may mean you have to distance yourself from these relationships in order to practice real self-care. Take the time to grieve the loss and remember that those who are healthy and whole themselves will support you. If you find yourself unable to disentangle from a particular relationship that you know is at odds with your real self-care practice, this can be an indicator that it's time to seek professional help.

I get that values are important, but it feels so good to me when I'm in productivity mode and checking goals off of my list. Is this bad?

Productivity becomes toxic when you haven't identified the values that are underneath your goals. This is why the Real Self-Care Compass is so powerful. With the Compass, your goals are secondary and your values—your **HOW** and your **WHY**—are primary. That doesn't mean we don't care about goals—being able to check tasks and milestones off a list is valuable. When you achieve a goal, you feel a sense of completion and resolution. It's not a bad thing to want and need that stability. It only becomes problematic when you lose track of *why* you care about the goal in the first place.

Remember Anita from Chapter 2, the small business owner and mom of three who was always on the lookout for the next organizational strategy or time-saving gadget? She was constantly focused on goals and gave lip service to the fact that her productivity obsession was in service of finding time for herself.

Yet that time for rest or recharging never came because she was addicted to her to-do list. This is the type of hyperfocus on productivity that we are trying to avoid—not productivity altogether.

YOUR VALUES VOCAB

Your quick reference when it comes to values

- Goals are tangibles to check off a list, while values are ongoing qualities of being—your **HOW** and your **WHY**.

- When making difficult decisions, turn inward to your values as opposed to looking outward to friends, colleagues, or relatives for answers.

- You'll know you're aligned with your values when your outsides match your insides.

- Avoiding fork-in-the-road moments can be a result of not being connected to your values.

- Digesting the good stuff in your life (past and present) makes room for more good stuff.

- It's normal for values to shift as you move through the seasons of your life.

Chapter 8

REAL SELF-CARE IS AN
ASSERTION OF POWER

CLAIMING WHAT'S YOURS
AND REMAKING THE SYSTEM

———

Sometimes people try to destroy you, precisely because
they recognize your power—not because they don't see
it, but because they see it and they don't want it to exist.

BELL HOOKS

I f, in the words of Audre Lorde, real self-care is a fight for self-
preservation and self-expression, then it follows that we need
practices to help us stay in touch with our own power. Systems
of oppression win by beating us down and stripping us of meaning and hope—they convince us that we are powerless against
them. Our work is to be unflinching in recasting our narrative
to one of power. In this way, we hold on to our agency, and can
implement change in our relationships, our workplaces, and our
systems.

Please don't mistake this for toxic positivity—a term that describes the whitewashing of hardship and negative feelings in

service of rushing to the positive. While comments like "every-thing happens for a reason" and "at least it wasn't more terrible" usually come from a place of good intention, not only are they not helpful to receive, they also dismiss the reality of loss, trauma, and the very real struggles of anyone who isn't in a privileged position in our society. Toxic positivity is the overwhelming urge to cast aside the struggle, pain, and losses you or others have experienced, and wrap it up into a tidy package of "I learned so much" or "Now I know better." The use of toxic positivity is yet another example of our discomfort with nuance and wanting to push forward instead of reflecting and feeling our feelings.

Not only is it *okay* to feel bad, it's also *useful*. In order to feel the good stuff in life, we also need to be able to feel the bad stuff. You can't have one without the other—otherwise you risk be-coming numb and apathetic. The reason for this is because the same parts of our brain that allow us to feel good feelings—like excitement, joy, and happiness—also enable us to experience bad feelings, like anger and grief. When you shut down your negative feelings, you're inadvertently shutting down your abil-ity to experience positive ones as well.

Here it can be helpful to understand the distinction between optimism and hope. It turns out that the common way we think about hope is all wrong—it isn't synonymous with optimism but a different skill altogether. Social scientist Arthur C. Brooks writes that hope means "believing you can make things better without distorting reality."[1] Researchers have found that while optimism is the sense that everything will be okay, people who are hopeful have the understanding that things may not be okay, but that they have agency to make things a little better for themselves or for others.[2] People who are hopeful don't pretend that bad things aren't happening—rather, they understand that to move forward we must integrate the good and the bad.

HOW PERSONAL CHOICES LEAD TO SYSTEMIC CHANGE

When I wrote my piece for *The New York Times*' "The Primal Scream" series about how what women were experiencing was *betrayal*, not burnout, a reader commented: "The problem seems to be that having inner peace and creating societal change are a tad at odds with each other." It makes sense for folks to have this perspective, and I did too. If the reason women are so desperate for wellness solutions is structural and systemic, it is reasonable to ask: What is the relationship between personal change and societal change?

A system changes only after a critical mass of individual people show up differently—in other words, *internal and individual changes made by many are a prerequisite for systemic change.* The two, individual and systemic, must occur together, but the good news is that they can form a positive feedback loop whereby individual changes inspire and give permission for more women to make their own internal shifts, which in turn puts pressure on the system to reorganize. In this way, even the marginalized among us can, in small ways, fight back against the system that has held us down.

Take for example Mikaleh, from Chapter 3, whose personal decision to take a leave of absence and care for her mental health led to organizational changes in her workplace. To take this step, Mikaleh had to do the work of real self-care: (1) recognize that it was up to her to set a boundary and reconcile the dialectic—she could be a stand-up employee *and* need to take time off for her health, she could love her father *and* ask her brothers to pitch in; (2) soften the internal narrative that she was weak and failing, as well as face her worries about retaliation, specifically around her identity as a Black woman in her workplace; (3) identify her values, which included taking care of her mental health; and (4) exercise her power, which meant exerting the rights her employer gave her.

We've seen this happen on the national stage as well. Over the short span of three months in 2021, two of the world's greatest athletes shocked the world by doing something extraordinary. Both Naomi Osaka, the highest-paid female athlete in the world, and Simone Biles, elite gymnast and gold medal winner, opted out: Osaka cited mental health struggles during the French Open and decided not to compete, and Biles withdrew from the team competition in the Tokyo Olympic Games after experiencing the twisties.

Here were two young Black women, powerful leaders at the top of their games, who had the power and clarity of mind to put themselves first—despite the fanfare, the pressure, and the possibility of more money and success. Both Osaka and Biles paid a price for making a hard choice—there were many who harshly criticized the decision to prioritize mental health. Yet many others lauded them as champions of self-care. Real self-care and saying no in the face of tremendous stakes does always come with a price, but that cost is less than what they would have paid if they had just kept going and martyred themselves.

I want to also draw attention to what we discussed in Chapter 1. The story of self-care coming into the public eye begins with some of the most marginalized people in our society—Black women in the 1960s. It's often those who are the most vulnerable who bear the burden of making change happen—because, as we discussed earlier, change rarely comes from the top down. So, it should not be lost on us that it's Black women who are showing us that self-care is not only possible, it's necessary. Particularly for folks who are marginalized in America, real self-care is a radical and crucial act to recover power from oppressive systems.

I can't claim to know about the internal processes of either of these female athletes, but as an onlooker, I find it looks remarkably similar to real self-care. Osaka and Biles offer powerful examples of how personal change, viewing yourself differently, and taking public action change the power structure of a system. For example, professional sports still have a long way to go in embracing the importance of athletes' mental health, but it's now part of the national conversation. After Biles made her decision, a patient shared with me that when speaking with friends about how impressed she was with Biles's choice, she disclosed her own struggle with depression. This conversation led to a friend in her circle asking for a recommendation for a therapist. This is *power*. When a person inside a system steps back and interacts with a long-standing system in a different way, she is serving as a lightning rod. In that act, they give permission for everyone else inside that system to question how it operates and if that mode of operating actually benefits them.

There is no doubt that the system all of us live in makes it tremendously difficult to make these choices in service of real self-care. In the following pages, I'm going to guide you through psychological techniques that will help you stay in touch with your power and help you remain hopeful in the face of adversity. These tools are designed to help you keep your eyes on that fact that real self-care is a fight against our systems. They will help you remember your agency in times when you feel beaten down or like it's impossible to exercise your choice.

LEAN INTO "BOTH, AND"

In the dark period after I had left the cult and was facing the terrifying prospect of returning to the medical world, I turned to a psychoanalyst mentor for advice and solace. Near the top of the list of questions I had for him was what it meant about my character that I had been in the group. I remember saying to him, "Am I the loser who dropped out of residency because she was a coward, fell for a scam, and ruined her life? Or am I the brave, forward-thinking woman who found something singular, and was courageous enough to follow my instinct?" He, being a psychoanalyst, answered my question with a question: "Is the knight on a chessboard a small, lifeless wooden object—or is he a powerful player that can change the stakes of the game?" The answer, of course: *He is both.*

After that conversation, it took me many years of psychoanalysis with my own therapist to fully internalize this paradox. In my case, the question that haunted me for a long time was, essentially: "Am I a *good* person or a *bad* person?" On one hand, I had not knowingly done anything wrong, but by being publicly involved with this group, I gave them legitimacy. For that, I felt shame and guilt. On the other hand, during that time in my life, I believed in the practice this group taught—orgasmic meditation. It was healing for me in profound ways—in my relationship with my body, in my understanding of myself, and in my relationship with the trauma I had experienced working in the medical system. Through my time there, I met a pioneering neuroscientists at the Rutgers orgasm lab, who took me under their wing. I spent two years learning what happens in the brain during orgasm for women. Now part of my clinical practice is taking care of women who suffer from genitopelvic pain conditions and sexual health issues.

When I left the cult, I was depressed, nearly suicidal, and scared. I ran back to the system I knew—medicine and academia. It was familiar and I needed shelter. But the lessons I learned from leaving the cult stayed with me. Moreover, because of my experience with extreme wellness, I developed an understanding of how wellness goes wrong, and what we can do to care for ourselves in a healthy, safe, and autonomous way.

Academic medicine is a high-demand system of its own—with a rigorous set of rules and expectations. This time, returning to my medical training, I was able to hold on to myself, set boundaries, and practice real self-care, while also maintaining a critical perspective on medicine and psychiatry. I knew the solutions other people gave me could never fit. I had to make hard choices. I had to prioritize myself. Over several years, my therapist gently helped me acknowledge this paradox and come to terms with my past. Would I be here now, with the voice I have and the belief and confidence in my own mission, if leaving the cult was not a part of my history? I'm not sure—but what I do know is that just like all of us, I contain good and bad parts.

What I'm speaking about here is the dialectic, which you may remember from Part I. Dialectical thinking refers to the ability to reconcile seemingly opposite points of view. In our polarized society, it's harder and harder to come by, which is also why it's so powerful. Dialectical behavioral therapy, which we discussed in Chapter 3, is based on the notion that change occurs when there is a resolution between opposite ends or conflicting ideas. In other words: "both, and."

The power of the dialectic is critical when it comes to real self-care. It's possible to move toward inner peace with your decisions *and* create societal change—these two are not at odds.

Take my patient Sonia, who felt guilt and shame for sending her kids to the babysitter on the weekends so she could catch up on work. She had to come to peace with her assertion of individual power within her family. It didn't lead to big changes in the moment, but ultimately Sonia's embrace of real self-care led to her husband asking for paternity leave at his small start-up. The company ended up initiating a paternity leave policy going forward, to attract and retain talent.

Inner peace and social change do not come without inner conflict. We are both the wooden figurine on the chessboard *and* powerful players with the capacity to change the game.

To Practice: Imagining Your Chessboard

Think back to the voices you identified in Chapter 6, when we were learning the skill of self-compassion—your optimist, your wise woman, and so on. Now think of a situation in which the knight on the chessboard metaphor applies to your life—perhaps a time when you felt powerless in the face of circumstances that were out of your control.

1. How would your optimist narrate the story? Your wise woman? Your quirky one?
2. Are there some universal truths that stand out to you in each of these retellings that apply no matter which voice is telling the story?

3. Imagine these different voices engaging with each other. Are there insights about your character or personality that stand out in each of these retellings? Some of these might apply across retellings, while some of them will likely be contradictory. That's okay.

When we look at ourselves and our situations from the lens of "both, and," we give ourselves the benefit of perspective. We recognize that there is rarely just one story, and we're able to see that more than one truth can be possible at the same time.

TURN UP YOUR COMPLEXITY

It naturally follows that after we focus on the dialectic, the path to remembering your power is to turn *up* the complexity of your story—not turn it down. Our culture has a way of flattening women's existence, and of viewing complexity and contradiction as a threat. Instead of seeing ourselves and our roles as one-dimensional, we can empower ourselves by reflecting on and embracing the alternative stories.

Several years ago, along with a colleague, I initiated a project with immigrant survivors of intimate partner violence.[3] We used a technique called testimonial therapy, in which survivors came together and shared their narratives of survival and strength. These women had been through horrific circumstances, not only in trying to seek refuge in the United States but also due to violence in their personal lives. In this process of sharing the good and the bad, the women no longer felt defined solely by their traumatic experiences. One survivor said that from the ashes of her prior relationship she carried the fact that "I was able to move forward, alone. . . . It took a lot of strength, yet I was able to do it." This survivor narrated her story as a journey of discovering the truth about a man who had betrayed her. Her testimony was marked by growth—she started off as a naive young woman and, at the end, she described a feeling of self-reliance and strength. This is not me waving a magic wand and saying that the trauma these survivors experienced was rightful or needed. Trauma is never deserved or needed. Instead, testimonial therapy is a modality that centers moving forward and finding sources of meaning and hope in the face of hardship.

Your Real Self-Care Compass can help with this, as you can apply your personal manifesto to various aspects of your life—your relationships, work, community—and bring your values forward in unexpected ways. For example, a friend of mine who works as a scientist and who deeply values adventure spent a recent sabbatical traveling internationally. Typically, scientists use their sabbaticals to write books or catch up on research projects—it's meant to be a time of concentrated work for pushing out peer-reviewed papers or gaining favor in the race for tenure. But my friend had spent the past few years burned out, facing a number of rejections and even considering leaving academics altogether. She viewed herself at the nadir of her career. So, from a place of desperation, she took a risk and followed a different path—she visited four countries over seven months and took her family along with her. She came back from her sab-batical refreshed and full of energy. Ultimately, she did not meet her department chair's expectations for academic productivity. One could think of that as a failure. Or you could say that be-cause of her time spent living life aligned with her values, she felt less conflicted about leaving academics for good and taking a job in the private sector (wherein she had more time off to travel and explore).

I suspect if you are reading this book, you have had some failures and losses, some memories in your past or even situa-tions in your present that make you wince when you think about them. It can be tempting to make those experiences our whole story—and social media, even our families and friends, might pull for hardship or trauma to define us. Yet if real self-care is about self-preservation and self-expression, it follows that we can find power in recasting our narratives. For example, I re-cently read a headline that said "Burned-Out Moms Gathered in a Field to Scream," and thought to myself, shouldn't the headline really be "Nation Abandons Mothers and They've Had Enough"? When we consider the alternative headlines and embrace the complexity of our stories, we are more likely to feel empowered.

To Practice: Owning Your Headline

When considering the headlines of our lives, it's often easier to start outside ourselves because it's easier to be generous to others and much harder to extend that generosity inward. With this practice, the goal is not to tell yourself that everything happens for a reason and all is perfect as it is (that's toxic positivity). Instead, our intent is to embrace the nuance and see if you can look back at a hard time in your life and find some nuggets of wisdom or truth.

1. Think of a friend who has gone through a tough time in life, whether it was due to a failure on their part or in relation to external circumstances like illness, divorce, or loss. Describe their story in terms of what was lost and the suffering they experienced.

2. Now think about how you could tell this story in a different way. What if instead of starting with the low point, you picked a different starting place? What other narratives are possible with this story? What hidden strengths lie inside your friend's low point in their life? Did you notice any positive changes in them that emerged as a result of this hardship? What meaning came out of the low point in their life?

3. Now go through these steps for yourself—identify a low or difficult moment in your own life and see if you can apply the same nuance and generosity toward yourself. Did you find meaning in unexpected places? How did your experience shape who you have become today?

Resisting the flattening of our stories helps us hold on to agency and power. It's one way to push back against our society's expectation that women conform to one stereotype or narrative.

Make a note of your answers for this exercise and keep them in a trusted place so that you can read over them when you are feeling low or stuck.

TRADE CYNICISM FOR AGENCY

You might be thinking, "This is all great for people who already have some power, like an author or a public figure, but what about the rest of us?" Let me reassure you that I see many tangible examples of real self-care in my clinical practice, working with patients who are dealing with the struggles of their daily lives, and are up against decisions that challenge them to the core.

Take my patient Lena, who worked as a video producer for a local TV station. Lena enjoyed her work, but she was woefully underpaid and undersupported. The TV station she worked at largely ignored employee complaints because they had won a series of prestigious awards in the industry. Lena felt like her hands were tied—if she spoke up about the lack of support she had, the station could easily let her go and find another producer who was champing at the bit to get their foot in the door. In one session she said, "What's the point of speaking up about my terrible working conditions? Nothing's going to change. I have no power here." Lena felt that no matter what she said, the status quo would prevail, and as such, it wasn't worth making a fuss.

Together, we worked through the process of real self-care, and Lena took a risk to set some boundaries with her work, such as no longer pulling all-nighters, and taking sick days when she needed them. She softened her self-talk, gave herself permission for self-compassion and got clear on her values. Lena was a creative individual and she was energized by the social justice programming that her network produced. She did not want to leave her job, but it was also not aligned with her values for Lena to keep getting the short end of the stick. So she began to ask questions—about what it would take for her boss to hire an assistant for her and about why her pay rate was so far below the market average for her experience and expertise. After a yearlong battle, Lena got an assistant. Perhaps even more powerful is that young women at the network saw Lena as an ally and began asking her for advice in their own careers. Ultimately, her advocacy for herself led to new policies being put in place so that producers had their costs reimbursed in a timely manner and several new assistants were hired for other folks at Lena's level. Lena is still negotiating for a raise for herself and advocating for a restructuring of her department to be more equitable for junior members, but these early wins helped her remember her agency in what is sure to be a long battle.

Practicing real self-care requires taking ownership of yourself back from the system that has held you down—whether that system is your family, your workplace, society writ large, or all of the above. If Lena had given in to cynicism, none of these changes would have occurred. Through her practice of real self-care, she was able to improve her own situation and the situations of those who would come after her.

To Practice: Planting the Seeds of Revolution

Real self-care is about changing our internal landscape so that we can go forth and exert power and agency in the outside world. I think of this as planting seeds of revolution—we are seeding the future for ourselves and for the next generation as well.

1. Make a list of recent situations or encounters that stand out to you as places where you have witnessed injustice or unfair practices.
2. Using your Real Self-Care Compass as a guide, reflect on where in your spheres of influence you might be able to assert agency and power for yourself or on behalf of others. This could take the form of asking questions about systems that are opaque in your workplace or starting a petition in your neighborhood.

The process of systemic change does not happen overnight. When we think about real self-care as a practice of planting the seeds of change, it helps us remember that this work is ongoing and blossoms in unexpected ways.

ESTABLISH HOPE AS A PRACTICE

At George Washington University, a group has operational-ized the practice of hope into what's called the Hope Modules.[4] Initially designed to support people who were going through severe illness, like cancer or chronic pain, the hope modules were expanded to apply to everyday people who are going through very difficult external stressors or adverse life circumstances. I was fortunate to receive training in this framework when I was a psychiatric resident and have seen it work for many patients. The gist of it is this: In order to cultivate hope, people need to activate one or more of four different types of coping skills:

- Problem-solving (i.e., jumping to a task or action that helps you move forward tangibly)
- Emotion regulation (i.e., reducing your in-the-moment stress level or feelings of discomfort)
- Activating a core identity (i.e., connecting with an individual or collective identity)
- Relational coping (i.e., connecting with mentors or important people in your life)

For example, when a patient of mine who has a medically complex child comes across the plethora of obstacles that her insurance puts up to getting coverage for medical care, she uses these skills: she makes a list of what she needs to get covered, she reminds herself that this work is hard and it's okay to take breaks, she goes to regular meetups with her church moms' group, and she spends time with a close friend who is also a mom of a special-needs kid. These hope-activating skills help her feel like she has some power.

She is not naive about her situation—it's a mess, and it's unfair that this is her fight, but at the same time she is able to recognize when her actions lead to progress for her daughter's health. She is careful not to take on the burden of trying to change the whole system—that would be impossible. But she uses these hope-building tools to prevent herself from becoming apathetic. In balancing the two extremes, that's where we hold on to hope—and with hope comes power.

To Practice: Identifying Your Hope-Building Skills

Everyone has the capacity to practice hope, whether you're an optimist or a pessimist. This exercise will help you identify which coping skills you already have and which come most naturally to you, so that you can continue to shore these up as you move forward in your real self-care practice.

1. Think of a recent experience in your life about which you feel crummy—it could be something going on in the world or something that's happened to you through no fault of your own, or an event that you feel ashamed or guilty about. Why did this situation make you feel so bad? If you can, try to remember the feelings that you experienced at the time.
2. Now remember what actions you took immediately after this event happened—in the hours, days, and weeks of the aftermath, how did you cope? Did you move into problem-solving and take specific actions like researching or collect-

ing more information? Or did you immediately reach out to a trusted friend or colleague (i.e., relational coping)? Perhaps your first instinct was to move into activating your core identity and connecting with your faith or church group.

3. If you can, get granular with your process. We often use a mix of all four coping skills in order to build hope for ourselves. And while for each of us there will be one or two that come most naturally, all of these tools are available to you in times of distress or hardship. If you found that you did not utilize any of them, reflect on if there is one that resonates most with you now that you can call up when you feel hopeless about change.

When faced with the litany of systemic constraints and failures, the practice of hope is the ultimate source of resistance because it's always available for us to practice. Make note of which hope-building skills come most naturally to you so that you can put them into practice during times of hardship or when you are starting to feel like you have no agency.

WHEN TO SEEK PROFESSIONAL HELP

It can be difficult to tell the difference between clinical depression or anxiety and the all-encompassing existential dread that comes with living through systemic oppression and the collapse of basic human rights. It's also possible to be experiencing both—despair over a world in which you feel powerless *and* a clinical mental health condition. In fact, when you're living through systemic failures and have less access to resources and support, you are more likely to suffer from a mental health condition. You can suffer from the effects of a deeply unjust society *and* benefit from treatment for a mental health condition. If you find yourself feeling consistently hopeless and unable to enjoy or take pleasure in any activities that typically cheer you up, this could be a sign that you're suffering from a clinical condition like depression. In some cases, extreme hopelessness can manifest as symptoms like going to bed at night and wishing you don't wake up in the morning or hoping that you are in a fatal accident. These types of thoughts are what we call passive suicidal ideation, and if you are experiencing them, seek care from a mental health professional.

PAY IT FORWARD

In the fall of 2021, something groundbreaking was happening. The US was coming up on nearly two years of being ravaged by a global pandemic. And for the first time in decades, the federal government had paid leave for caregivers and new parents on the table in the form of the Build Back Better Act. In the initial iteration of this legislation, Congress proposed twelve weeks of paid parental leave. And then, as quickly as we cheered, paid leave was removed from the bill due to opposition from several senators.

Women and mothers were furious. So they took to the streets—literally. Thousands of mothers showed up at the steps of our nation's capitol, in the rain, to demand that paid leave be brought back into the proposed legislation. Grassroots movements popped up all over the country. On social media, a coalition of advocates and leaders came together, and we called ourselves the Chamber of Mothers. Nearly overnight a movement of ten thousand women came together to take action.

Due to the work of new advocates and groups that have been working on this issue for decades, lawmakers put paid leave back into the legislation—albeit at four weeks instead of twelve. What was striking to me about this movement is that many of the women who signed up, donated, and showed up in the rain were done having children. They were not going to personally benefit from a federal leave policy. But they were willing to donate their time, energy, and money for others who would benefit. They were paying it forward. Moreover, the logistics around this movement took into account the fact that people who had the privilege to show up to protest and to organize had resources—such as childcare or support at home—so that they could get on a bus to Washington, DC. Groups organized donation campaigns to pay for childcare so that women who did not have those choices could come and fight for this cause.

Another phrase for the collectivism of paying it forward is *community care*. I believe that community care is a by-product of real self-care—for with power comes responsibility. Angela

Garbes, author of *Essential Labor: Mothering as Social Change*, talks about the fact that minority communities have been engaging in community care for centuries—it's how folks who do not have access to systemic resources survive: neighborhood libraries, trading off playdates, carpooling to work. Angela has said, "One of the central pieces of community is decentering yourself . . . sometimes you are the person who is giving, you are not always the person receiving."[5] Ultimately, the work of real self-care is about changing our relationships with ourselves, and, in turn, what naturally follows such internal change is a reorganizing of larger systems. In order for this reorganization to be equitable for the women who are most disadvantaged, those of us who hold privilege must share the power we build through real self-care. This might mean giving up opportunities, convenience, or status so that resources can be distributed to women who are lacking.

In my own life, when I made the decision to leave full-time academic work, I recognized there were privileges involved with being able to make that choice. Now I hold office hours for physicians and trainees who are looking to start their own practices, to write articles and books for a nonscientific community, or to explore entrepreneurship. It's one small way that I can pay it forward to the next generation of physician creatives who are building careers outside of the traditional framework.

To Practice: Cultivating Community Care

As you now know, real self-care has the power to change the systems that we live and work inside. When we think about community care, it's helpful to understand the areas of your life wherein you have experienced oppression and the areas of your life in which you hold privilege. When you make this explicit, it's easier to pay it forward. Ask yourself the following questions to assess how privilege and oppression show up in your own life.

1. What privileges or advantages do I hold (e.g., partnered or married, American citizen, cisgender, light skin)?
2. What factors put me at risk for oppression (e.g., lack of financial resources, single parent, disabled, coming from a historically marginalized or oppressed identity group)?
3. What is easy and simple for me that is harder for other people?
4. What is one way I can be generous in my personal life?
5. What is one way I can be generous in my professional life?

Reflecting on these questions is not meant to induce guilt or shame. Instead, I'm gently proposing that you spend time reflecting on the areas of your life in which you can afford to be generous. Keep in mind that community care does not need to be grand, sweeping gestures—it can be dropping off dinner to a neighbor whom you don't know but who just had a baby, or reaching out to a younger colleague whom you have nothing in common with to grab coffee.

———

The reality of living as a woman in America means that our fight for real self-care never ends. You could think of this as a failure, or you could embrace it for what it is—looking truth in the eye: we are living in the gray space of "both, and."

For example, at the time of writing this book, federal paid leave policy has stalled and reproductive and human rights have been rolled back in the United States. I'm not sure where legislation supporting caregivers or other progressive causes will be when you read these lines. That said, focusing on the results of specific legislation misses the point. Remember our chessboard: We could sink in despair over policy and advocacy failures. Or we could recognize that the energy and collective power that was harnessed by individuals in 2021 has led to real and tangible changes at the state level and in the corporate sector. In Maryland and Delaware, for example, state legislators passed paid leave policies in 2022. We saw huge multinational corporations come out with progressive family leave policies—not just for parents, but for all caregivers—and policies for mental health leave and other benefits. Of course, there is much more work to be done (for example, it's not sustainable to depend on corporate America to provide services and protections that should come from our government), *and* recognizing individual and collective agency is a powerful source of hope.

Audre Lorde said, "Your power is relative, but it is real. And if you do not learn to use it, it will be used against you, and me, and our children. Change did not begin with you, and it will not end with you, but what you do with your life is an absolutely vital piece of that chain."[6] Especially in times of trauma at the national and international levels, our power comes from the practice of hope and focusing, unflinchingly, on the fact that our agency comes from the collective will to empower ourselves. We do this through embracing the complexity of ourselves and others, and by lifting up those of us who are the most vulnerable.

SOUNDS GREAT, BUT . . .

There are aspects of my life where I feel really privileged (I have a stable job, I have a partner, I'm in good health) but then other aspects where I know I've been disadvantaged (I'm a woman of color). How do I know if I'm supposed to be "giving back" or "getting help"?

Privilege and oppression are not binary. Both occur across a spectrum. This is another example of how "both, and" thinking helps us see the nuance of our situations. For example, as this question suggests, there may be aspects of your life wherein you have resources and privilege—perhaps you have access to a top education or you are in a position of power in your workplace. On the other hand, there might be aspects of your identity or your personal history that put you at a disadvantage—like being an immigrant or living with a disability. Both of these can be true at the same time, and this means that there may be some circumstances in which you have more to give and can lend a helping hand, while there are others in which you could benefit from added help.

What if treating myself and giving myself breaks is something that I really enjoy? Do I need to feel guilty that I'm not advocating for a greater cause or doing something bigger for the system?

The purpose of real self-care is not to induce guilt or shame. Neither feeling is a helpful motivator. And especially in the past few years, it's true that more and more people have turned to "treat yourself" practices simply to get through the day. When the world feels out of control, if you have the means, giving yourself treats—whether it's a chocolate bar or going out for a manicure—can be a way to exert agency. You set your sights on a task and complete it—this feels good. Instead of feeling guilty about it, is it possible to channel the relief that you feel into taking positive action for someone who has less than you? Can you send an email providing positive feedback for a colleague who is a person of color? Can you spare five minutes to sign a letter of support for an elected official whose platform is aligned with your values?

Research tells us that prosocial behavior—that is, taking action that benefits others—is not only good for the people you are helping, it also improves the emotional well-being of the person who is doing the helping.[7] Again, the goal here is not to flagellate ourselves into change, but instead to reconsider how each of us can exert small amounts of agency and power in the wider system.

YOUR POWER PROGRAM

Your quick list when it comes to remembering your power

- Embracing "both, and" as opposed to "either, or" keeps you connected to your power.

- Acknowledging bad feelings is not a waste of time; it's the path you must take to practice hope and, in turn, gain power.

- It's not your job to change the whole system; it's your job to stay in touch with your agency.

- When you flatten your story (or the stories of others), you give up power.

- Giving back when you have power generates more power for everyone else.

- Hope is not something you have or don't have; it's a skill to build.

CONCLUSION

The path that led me to writing this book started with feeling existentially disillusioned with psychiatry. As a young physician, I was taught that our patients are broken and in need of fixing. Yet what I saw were policies and social structures that held my patients down. It was obvious to me that medication was not going to fix these external problems, and I felt betrayed by a medical establishment that did nothing to teach me how to help my patients struggling in a world that was not built for them. My disillusionment with psychiatry led me down the rabbit hole of faux self-care.

I think about what I've learned in the past decade of my life, recovering from the aftermath of extreme wellness, and the first image that comes to mind is of Yayoi Kusama—an iconic Japanese artist who suffers from schizophrenia. At the age of ten, living in a rural village, Kusama began to experience visual hallucinations, in the form of dots, flowers, and repetitive images. She pursued her art, which was unheard of for a woman in 1950s Japan, let alone a woman with serious mental illness. Kusama has gone on, against all odds, to be considered the most successful female artist alive. Her work is based in feminism and surrealism. Visiting one of the many Kusama exhibits that have taken the world by storm is like taking a trip into the artist's mind—unique, powerful, and full of life. She now lives in a Tokyo psychiatric hospital, where she has built her own art studio. Auction houses have sold more than $500 million worth of her art in the past decade.

When I consider Kusama, the word *broken* is the furthest thing from my mind.

Instead, I know that power comes from some of life's most devastating hardships. Our strength is in taking ownership of the pain, allowing ourselves to feel it as such, *and* continuing to move forward despite the suffering. Illness, hardship, trauma, loss—none of it is a life sentence. It's the most painful things about ourselves that have the capacity to bring out the most brilliance.

I feel hope, not only because of stories like Yayoi's, but because of what I hear from my patients. There is a clarity with which they know, deeply, that the status quo is not working. They are bringing the systemic issues—of income inequality, unpaid labor, and social oppression—into the therapy room like never before. They understand that they are not broken or in need of fixing; it's our social fabric that needs repair. This is the definition of progress—when we see what's happening in front of us clearly and without distortion.

The work of real self-care is to hold hope and pain together. As women, we are perpetually living at the precipice—grappling to hold on to ourselves inside a storm that is raging for us to let go and give up. Faux self-care keeps us treading water—worn down, tired, and hopeless. Real self-care is your life raft. And when enough of us internalize real self-care, the tide finally shifts, and we wake up to the power that's possible.

Acknowledgments

I have many people to thank—not only for the physical existence of this book but also for the emotional support that enabled me to reach a place in my life such that I could write it.

First and foremost, thank you to my patients for giving me the honor of walking your path with you. I can only be here because of the people who have trusted me with their stories.

I'm also grateful for the expertise of those who came before me. Winnicott said, "It is not possible to be original except on the basis of tradition." I'm able to share what I have because of the clinicians, researchers, activists, and public intellectuals who have been doing the painstaking work of advocating for women's mental health and intersectional feminism long before my time.

Writing a book is an exercise in self-discipline. I imagined what my killjoys would say about me. I worried that I was not getting it right. The fact that I carried on and was able to complete a project this vast is largely because I was fortunate to find a team of smart, kind, and forward-thinking women in the publishing industry to help me bring *Real Self-Care* into the world.

My agent, Rachel Sussman—you've walked this path with me since 2019 and have never doubted my vision. Part agent, part editor, part therapist—a day doesn't go by without me thanking my lucky stars that you took a risk with me. You're in the weeds with me in a way that is deeply kind and pretty much unheard of for an agent. You got me through writing a book while I was pregnant! For that, at least, you deserve an award. Thank you for always answering all of my many, many questions, for advising me on the all the thorny bits, for smoothing out my neurosis—and, most of all, for believing in me and my work.

My first editor, Jenna Free—my book doula. Without you this book would still be a cloud of feelings in my nervous system. Thank you for holding my thoughts with such compassion, and for helping me understand how my ideas connected, even when I felt like it was too hard (like when I was in the first trimester and wanted to dump this manuscript in the trash). I'm especially grateful for how you held my hand through the writing of the more personal bits of this book.

Thank you to my best-in-class team at Penguin Life. Meg Leder, my editor extraordinaire—every note you gave me made *Real Self-Care* more meaningful and clear. Your editorial eye has undoubtedly made this book a thousand times more useful than it would have been without you. Besides your unparalleled editing skill, thank you for allowing me to spend *so* much time talking about our depressingly *crappy* systems while also writing a self-help book! Shelby Meizlik, Lydia Hirt, Sabila Khan, and the rest of the Penguin Life team—thank you for *getting it* immediately, and for working so hard to spread the message of *Real Self-Care* far and wide.

Thank you to Anna Argenio, Najma Finlay, Lydia Weigel, Claire Busy, and the whole team at Cornerstone in the UK for your excitement and energy to bring *Real Self-Care* to an international audience. Anna, your enthusiasm for *Real Self-Care* is quite literally contagious—the way you've rallied behind me and my message, and the thoughtfulness you brought to the book editorially and beyond, has been an utter joy for me.

Thank you to Lauren Cerand—we're just getting started and I already feel deeply seen by you. I am so appreciative of the thoughtfulness and keen attention you bring.

There have been so many colleagues and advisers from various points in my life, who along the way championed me and my work. How does one live up to the pressure of writing a complete list of everyone to thank without having a nervous breakdown? I will do my best to keep this list specific to *Real Self-Care* and my writing: I'm hugely grateful to Jess Grose, Farah Miller, Melonyce McAfee, and the entire *New York Times* Parenting team who first gave me the privilege of channeling my rage into something more. Drew Ramsey, your generosity is rare—having you as my fellow psychiatrist guide has given me permission to dream about what's possible. Eve Rodsky, thank you for cheering me every step of the way with this book. Robert Solomon, thank

you for answering all of my questions, and please don't stop reminding me to have fun. Salman Akhtar, thank you for holding
a candle for me in the most difficult moment of my life—what
you taught me informs this book at a deep level.

I'm enormously grateful to Martha Beck for our conversation
about culture, koans, and Martyr Mode.

Conversations and kinship with the following change-making
women inspired and energized me while I was writing this book
and preparing to launch it into the world: Erin Erenberg, Cassie
Shortsleeve, Daphne Delvaux, Alexis Barad-Cutler, Raena Boston,
Kelsey Lucas, Cait Zogby, Dana Suskind, Rebecca Lehrer, Avni
Patel Thompson, Brigid Schulte, Hitha Palepu, Heather Irobunda,
Vania Manipod, Saumya Dave, Hina Talib, Kelly Fradin, Arghavan
Salles, Jill Grimes, Mia Clarke, Amy Barnhorst, Kaz Nelson, and
Nan Wise.

Rebecca Fernandez and your team at VOKSEE, thank you for
executing the vision I had for my website so beautifully.

Josh Zimmerman, thank you for always bringing me back to
my mission. Wendy Karlyn, thank you bringing me into new
rooms and championing me. Jessi Gold, I'm grateful for the
memes and the knowing. Lauren Smith Brody, thank you for
being a whip-smart sounding board on book writing, media, and
motherhood. Janna Meyrowitz Turner, my notes from our chats
live in a special file folder—you're brilliant. Pandora Sykes, thank
you for the delicious conversations, and I hope for many more
to come. Monisha Vasa, my nervous system calms when I see
your face—thank you for the caring you bring. Steve Steury, for

the walks and the dinners. Peter Polatin, for reminding me to think big.

I am endlessly grateful to Lisa Catapano, a mentor whom I'm now fortunate to call a friend—thank you for taking a chance on me in 2014 and for being in my corner through so many transitions.

Thank you to Windy Johnson for joyfully pitching in to help where I needed it and making sure my patients did not get lost while I was on maternity leave. And thank you to Nicole Perras for making it possible for me to take a maternity leave from my practice.

I'm grateful for the group of women physicians who came together with me on Zoom when the pandemic started and who are still going strong—Diana, Vero, Pooja, Sural, Marwa, Shannon, Stephanie, Michelle—thank you for being on my team.

Alexis, Nelia, Abby, Becca, Meagan, Amanda, Angie, Ashley, Amy, Lindsay, and Sydnia—I still can't believe you invited me to sit at your table.

Thank you to Magera Holton, Gio Fernandez-Kincade, Andi Ruda, Manuel Toscano, Murray Indick, Perry Lane, Bethany Saltman, Marta Perez, and Jennifer Lincoln, for all you've brought to Gemma. A special thank-you to Astrid Storey for your brilliant operations brain.

Lucy Hutner, we came into each other's lives at a very special time and found out just how much we have to learn from each other. I'm so grateful for the acceptance and understanding that you shine on me.

Kali Cyrus, you proved to me that we can make forever friends past age thirty. It's an honor to create the map of how to be a psychiatrist who colors outside the lines with you. Thank you for being a fellow big dreamer with me.

I would not be where I am in my life without the love and acceptance of my closest lifelong friends, who stuck with me through all of the storms. Puja, Denise, Mary, and Molly: You get me like no one else. Our friendship is one of the things I am most deeply proud of. You've jumped on a plane for me, you've been up in the middle of the night having utterly pointless conversations with me, you've been my first phone call when things fall apart, you've thrown me more than one party that I tried very hard not to attend, you've workshopped titles and book covers, you've made my baby registry because I was too busy writing this book. Thank you for loving me, all of me. Xing, Danielle, and Diane—my cheer squad—I'm so grateful for our twenty-plus years and counting.

I'm grateful to Brigette, our postpartum doula, who showed me the power of reliable and dependable childcare. Thank you for being with us on those nights I was crying over breastfeeding. The last edits on this manuscript came together because of your steadfast support of our family.

Christie, my psychoanalyst and therapist, who has been with me through the most important seasons of my life thus far: I faced my ambivalence about being called an "expert" and my conflict about my ambition while in your hands. I also graduated residency, found a life partner, adopted two cats, moved across the country, and had a baby. Thank you for allowing me to take risks, for never judging my impulses, and, most of all, for helping me grow up. There's no question in my mind that this book would not exist without you.

I'm grateful to my mother-in-law, Susan, and my sister-in-law, Samantha, whose support during my pregnancy and the birth of our son was instrumental in me being able to write this book. Thank you to Kevin, DJ, and Ashley for being my hype-squad, and to Steve and Molly for being our people.

I owe much more than I know to my roots in India. To the Shampur women in Bangalore, I have nothing but gratitude for our lineage.

Thank you to my sister, Deepa. Being the little sister of a psychiatrist is not an easy job and you live up to the challenge with humor, sass, and a fair bit of emo. Thanks for being my fiercest fan (and for showing me how to make a Reel). Love you.

To my parents—this book is the result of a decade of work to understand, reflect, and stay connected. It's not been easy, and we don't always get it right, but we have come such a long way and for that I am proud of us and grateful. Thank you for standing by my side through it all and for supporting me in my most grand dream of all—to become me.

Finally, my biggest thank-you goes to my partner, Justin. For believing in me and my big dreams without hesitation. For standing by my side when I decided to leave my full-time academic job and set out on an unknown path. For being the first reader and editor of all my drafts. For making sure I'm always fed and watered and that we have a home and that somebody checks the mail. For giving me all of those damn IVF injections. For loving Kiran, Kitty, and Fifi like you do. For teaching me so much of what I know about commitment, connection, and safety.

And, Kiran, it will be many years before you read this book (if you ever do?). I wrote it while you were growing into a human being inside me. Your arrival in the world is inextricably tied to real self-care, and for that, I am grateful, humbled, and filled with wonder.

Appendix 1

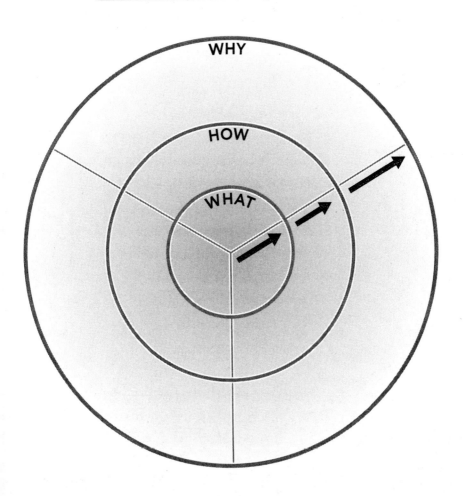

THE REAL SELF-CARE COMPASS

WHY

HOW

WHAT

Appendix 2

REAL SELF-CARE EXERCISES GUIDE

Principle I. Real self-care requires setting boundaries and moving past guilt

Principle II. Real self-care means treating yourself with compassion

Principle III. Real self-care brings you closer to yourself

To Practice: Your Birthday Dinner—page 173

To Practice: What I Know to Be True for Me—page 181

To Practice: Letting Yourself Have the Good Stuff—page 185

Principle IV: Real self-care is an assertion of power

To Practice: Imagining Your Chessboard—page 209

To Practice: Owning Your Headline—page 212

To Practice: Planting the Seeds of Revolution—page 216

To Practice: Identifying Your Hope-Building Skills—page 218

To Practice: Cultivating Community Care—page 223

The Real Self-Care Thermometer—page 86

The Real Self-Care Compass—page 188

Appendix 3

RESOURCES FOR SEEKING PROFESSIONAL HELP

For help finding a mental health professional (like a psychiatrist or a psychologist), some of the best resources include:

- Ask your primary care provider if they have mental health professionals that they refer to and like, and if they can share names with you.

- Many mental health professionals have a profile on psychology today.com, which is a nationwide resource. On their profiles, clinicians will post their areas of specialization, whether they take insurance, and if they are accepting new patients or clients. You can search *Psychology Today* based on specific identities as well—such as Native American or queer- and trans-sensitive care.

- If you have someone in your life whom you trust who has been in therapy or sees a mental health professional, reaching out to them can be helpful. They can give you the name of their therapist or ask their therapist for names of local clinicians. Word of mouth is often a helpful way to find a good therapist.

- If you are in the pregnancy or postpartum period, or dealing with mental health issues related to motherhood, Postpartum Support

International is an organization with chapters in every US state. They also have an online directory of clinicians who specialize in women's mental health at the website postpartum.net. One of their resources, in partnership with HRSA, is a 24-7 national maternal mental health hotline, staffed by mental health professionals who speak English and Spanish (1-833-9-HELP4MOMS).

- If you are dealing with pregnancy or perinatal loss, or struggling with mental health related to infertility, RESOLVE: the National Infertility Association has a list of support groups and therapists who specialize in this field (resolve.org).

If you are from a group that has historically been oppressed and is currently marginalized, there are several organizations through which to find a mental health professional who specializes in working with minority identities:

- If you are a Black woman: Therapy for Black Girls: therapyforblackgirls.com

- If you are a Latinx person: Latinx Therapy: latinxtherapy.com; Therapy for Latinx: therapyforlatinx.com

- If you are South Asian: South Asian Therapists.org: southasiantherapists.org

- If you identify as queer or trans and are a person of color: the National Queer & Trans Therapists of Color Network: nqttcn.com

- If you are parenting as an LGBTQ+ person: Rainbow Families: rainbowfamilies.org

If you are having a psychiatric emergency or are in crisis, please call the 988 Suicide & Crisis Lifeline at 988, go to the nearest ER, or call 911.

HOW DO YOU KNOW IF THE THERAPIST OR PSYCHIATRIST THAT YOU'RE SEEING IS A GOOD ONE?

The most important indicator of success in a therapy relationship is the therapeutic alliance—the relationship between therapist and patient. It follows that finding the right mental health professional is a bit like dating—fit matters. It's a good idea to conduct a few interviews and see who you get a good feeling from. It can sometimes take a couple of sessions to see if someone is the right fit for you.

Notice how your therapist responds to feedback—are they open and curious and does it deepen the conversation when you share feedback, or do they become defensive and critical? A good therapist will take your concerns seriously and want to work with you to understand how the relationship can improve. This means that it's your job to be open about what's working and what's not. Therapy is a collaborative process. If your therapist is judgmental or defensive, they might not be the best fit for you.

Notes

A WORD ON IDENTITY, PRIVILEGE, AND SYSTEMS OF OPPRESSION

1. Jordan Kisner, "The Lockdown Showed How the Economy Exploits Women. She Already Knew," *New York Times*, February 17, 2021, nytimes.com/2021/02 /17/magazine/waged-housework.html.

CHAPTER 1: EMPTY CALORIES: FAUX SELF-CARE HASN'T SAVED US

1. "2012 Stress in America: Stress by Gender," accessed July 22, 2022, apa.org /news/press/releases/stress/2012/gender.
2. Nancy Beauregard et al., "Gendered Pathways to Burnout: Results from the SALVEO," *Annals of Work Exposures and Health* 62, no. 4 (May 2018): 426–37.
3. Olivia Remes et al., "A Systematic Review of Reviews on the Prevalence of Anxiety Disorders in Adult Populations," accessed July 22, 2022, doi.org /10.1002/brb3.497; Paul R. Albert, "Why Is Depression More Prevalent in Women?" *Journal of Psychiatry and Neuroscience* 40, no. 4 (July 2015): 219–21.
4. "Antidepressant Use among Adults: United States, 2015–2018," NCHS Data Brief no. 377, September 2020.
5. "Wellness Industry Statistics & Facts," Global Wellness Institute, accessed October 17, 2022, globalwellnessinstitute.org/press-room/statistics-and-facts.
6. Audre Lorde, *A Burst of Light* (Ithaca, NY: Firebrand Books, 1988).
7. Angela A. Richard et al., "Delineation of Self-Care and Associated Concepts," *Journal of Nursing Scholarship* 43, no. 3 (September 2011): 255–64.
8. Barbara Riegel and Debra K. Moser, "Self-Care: An Update on the State of the Science One Decade Later," *Journal of Cardiovascular Nursing* 33, no. 5 (September/October 2018): 404–7.
9. Kisner, Jordan. "The Politics of Conspicuous Displays of Self-Care," *New Yorker*, March 14, 2017.
10. Greg McKeown, *Effortless* (New York: Currency, 2021).

CHAPTER 2: WHY IT'S HARD TO RESIST THE SEDUCTION: THE WAYS WE TURN TO FAUX SELF-CARE

1. "News Release: Wellness Tourism Association Releases Findings from First Wellness Travel Survey," Wellness Tourism Association, accessed July 22, 2022, old.wellnesstourismassociation.org/wellness-tourism-association-releases -findings-first-wellness-travel-survey.

2. Caroline Mortimer, "Women Criticise Themselves an Average of Eight Times a Day, Study Says," *Independent*, January 4, 2016, independent.co.uk/life-style /health-and-families/health-news/women-criticise-themselves-an-average-of -eight-times-a-day-study-says-a6796286.html.

3. Suniya S. Luthar and Lucia Ciciolla, "Who Mothers Mommy? Factors That Contribute to Mothers' Well-Being," *Developmental Psychology* 51, no. 12 (December 2015): 1812–23.

4. Anna Sutton, "Living the Good Life: A Meta-Analysis of Authenticity, Well-being and Engagement," *Personality and Individual Differences* 153 (January 15, 2022), sciencedirect.com/science/article/pii/S019188691930577X.

CHAPTER 3: THE GAME IS RIGGED: YOU'RE NOT THE PROBLEM

1. Petra Persson and Maya Rossin-Slater, "When Dad Can Stay Home: Fathers' Workplace Flexibility and Maternal Health," working paper no. 3928, January 22, 2021, gsb.stanford.edu/faculty-research/working-papers/when-dad-can-stay -home-fathers-workplace-flexibility-maternal.

2. Richard J. Petts et al., "Paid Paternity Leave-Taking in the United States," *Community, Work & Family* 23 no. 2 (July 17, 2017), doi.org/10.1080/13668803.2018.1471589.

3. Anne Helen Petersen, "From Burnout to Radicalization," *Culture Study* (blog), August 6, 2021, annehelen.substack.com/p/from-burnout-to-radicalization.

4. Caitlyn Collins et al., "COVID-19 and the Gender Gap in Work Hours," *Gender, Work, & Organization* 28, no. S1 (January 2021): 101–12.

5. Gretchen Livingston and Deja Thomas, "Among 41 Countries, Only US Lacks Paid Parental Leave," Pew Research Center, December 16, 2019, pewresearch .org/fact-tank/2019/12/16/u-s-lacks-mandated-paid-parental-leave.

6. Rasheed Malik, "Working Families Are Spending Big on Childcare," Center for American Progress, June 20, 2019, americanprogress.org/article/working-families -spending-big-money-child-care.

7. Meg Conley, "Motherhood in America Is a Multilevel Marketing Scheme," *Gen*, December 7, 2020, gen.medium.com/motherhood-in-america-is-a-multilevel -marketing-scheme-f4ec1f536b04.

8. Silvia Federici, *Re-Enchanting the World: Feminism and the Politics of the Commons* (Oakland, CA: PM Press, 2019).

9. Allison Daminger, "The Cognitive Dimension of Household Labor," *American Sociological Review* 84, no. 4 (July 9, 2019), journals.sagepub.com/doi/10.1177 /0003122419859007.

10. Lucia Ciciolla et al., "Invisible Household Labor and Ramifications for Adjustment: Mothers as Captains of Households," *Sex Roles* 81, no. 7–8 (October 2019): 1–20.
11. Gloria Steinem, *Outrageous Acts and Everyday Rebellions* (New York: Holt, 1983).
12. Dr. Martha Beck's work on how women navigate the contradictions in our culture deeply informs my view of women's mental health. In her 1997 book, *The Breaking Point: Why Women Fall Apart and How They Can Re-create Their Lives*, Dr. Beck presents the results of her sociological studies looking at women who come to crisis points in their lives, and how they resolve conflicts with culture.
13. Pooja Lakshmin, "Mothers Don't Have to Be Martyrs," *New York Times*, May 5, 2020, nytimes.com/2020/05/05/parenting/mothers-not-martyrs.html.
14. Jennifer L. Barkin et al., "The Role of Maternal Self-Care in New Motherhood," *Midwifery* 29, no. 9 (September 2013): 1050–5.
15. Albert Einstein, "Atomic Education Urged by Einstein," *New York Times*, May 25, 1946.
16. Dialectical behavior therapy, or DBT, is a type of psychotherapy that focuses on four areas of skills building: mindfulness, distress tolerance, emotion regulation, and interpersonal effectiveness. It's a type of therapy that can be helpful for several different psychiatric conditions, including depression, eating disorders, PTSD, substance abuse, and chronic suicidal ideation. DBT is strongly influenced by the concept of the dialectic, and encourages people to hold seemingly opposing perspectives at once.
17. Audre Lorde, *A Burst of Light* (Ithaca, NY: Firebrand Books, 1988).
18. Brigid Schulte, "Providing Care Changes Men," New America, accessed July 22, 2022, newamerica.org/better-life-lab/reports/providing-care-changes-men /executive-summary.
19. Interview with Brigid Schulte, October 15, 2021.

CHAPTER 4: TAKING BACK THE REINS:
THE FOUR PRINCIPLES OF REAL SELF-CARE

1. R. M. Ryan et al., "On Happiness and Human Potentials: A Review of Research on Hedonic and Eudaimonic Well-Being," *Annual Review of Psychology* 52 (2001): 141–66.
2. A. D. Turner et al., "Is Purpose in Life Associated with Less Sleep Disturbance in Older Adults?" *Sleep Science Practice* 1, no. 14 (2017).
3. Andrew Steptoe et al., "Subjective Wellbeing, Health, and Ageing," *Lancet* 385, no. 9968 (February 4, 2015): 640–8.
4. Barbara L. Frederickson et al., "A Functional Genomic Perspective on Human Well-being," *PNAS* 110, no. 33 (July 29, 2013): 13684–9, pnas.org/doi/10.1073 /pnas.1305419110.
5. Acceptance and commitment therapy (ACT) was developed by Steven Hayes, PhD, a clinical psychologist. ACT is a form of evidence-based psychotherapy

that is built on the broad technique of psychological flexibility, or the ability to develop a flexible relationship with your mind. ACT teaches patients how to accept difficult thoughts and feelings as opposed to fighting against them, and to prioritize taking committed actions that lead to a rich and meaningful life.

6. Brené Brown, "The Power of Vulnerability," TEDx Houston, accessed July 22, 2022, ted.com/talks/brene_brown_the_power_of_vulnerability/transcript.

CHAPTER 5: REAL SELF-CARE REQUIRES BOUNDARIES: MOVING PAST GUILT

1. Nedra Glover Tawwab, *Set Boundaries, Find Peace: A Guide to Reclaiming Yourself* (New York: TarcherPerigee, 2021).

2. If you have a history of traumatic or abusive relationships (either in the family you grew up in or as an adult), the way your body responds to requests might be confusing. There may be certain relationships or situations that initially feel like a yes but, in the aftermath, leave you feeling bad or ashamed. Note that for you, it might feel unsafe to communicate your boundaries. For those of you who would like to go deeper into untangling these responses and learn more about how trauma can impact relationships, Melody Beattie's *Beyond Codependency: And Getting Better All the Time* is an excellent resource for diving deeper into healing from traumatic or codependent relationships.

3. *Fair Play: A Game-Changing Solution for When You Have Too Much to Do (and More Life to Live)* outlines an organization system developed by Eve Rodsky. Eve emphasizes clarifying the CPE (Conception, Planning, and Execution) for each task that's involved in managing a household. This book is a great starting point for examining how decisions get made in your household, and who is responsible for planning and executing these decisions.

CHAPTER 6: REAL SELF-CARE MEANS TREATING YOURSELF WITH COMPASSION: PERMISSION TO BE GOOD ENOUGH

1. Kristin D. Neff, "The Role of Self-Compassion in Development: A Healthier Way to Relate to Oneself," *Human Development* 52, no. 4 (June 2009): 211–4.

2. Liliana Pedro et al., "Self-Criticism, Negative Automatic Thoughts and Postpartum Depressive Symptoms: The Buffering Effect of Self-compassion," *Journal of Reproductive and Infant Psychology* 37, no. 5 (April 5, 2019): 539–53, doi.org/10.1080/02646838.2019.1597969.

3. Pooja Lakshmin, "Mothers Don't Have to Be Martyrs," *New York Times*, May 5, 2020, nytimes.com/2020/05/05/parenting/mothers-not-martyrs.html.

4. Brené Brown, "Listening to Shame," TED 2012, accessed July 22, 2022, ted.com/talks/brene_brown_listening_to_shame.

5. Historical records suggest the concept of "the good enough mother" originally came from Winnicott's second wife, Clare Winnicott. Yet Donald Winnicott is frequently credited with this theory and the term.

6. Jennifer Senior, "It's Your Friends Who Break Your Heart," *Atlantic*, March 2022, theatlantic.com/magazine/archive/2022/03/why-we-lose-friends-aging-happiness /621305.

7. Jessica Grose, "Practicing Self-Care in Uncertain Times," *New York Times*, November 4, 2020, nytimes.com/2020/11/04/parenting/exhaustion-burnout-rest .html.

CHAPTER 7: REAL SELF-CARE BRINGS YOU CLOSER TO YOURSELF: BUILDING YOUR REAL SELF-CARE COMPASS

1. Russ Harris, *ACT Made Simple: A Quick Start Guide to ACT Basics and Beyond* (Oakland, CA: New Harbinger, 2009).

2. Daniel B. M. Haun et al., "Children Conform to the Behavior of Peers; Other Great Apes Stick with What They Know," *Psychological Science* 25, no. 12 (December 2014): 2160–7.

3. Martha Beck, *The Way of Integrity: Finding the Path to Your True Self* (New York: Open Field, 2021).

4. Caroline Gregoire, "Jack Kornfield on Gratitude and Mindfulness," *Greater Good Magazine*, May 14, 2019, greatergood.berkeley.edu/article/item/jack_kornfield _on_gratitude_and_mindfulness.

CHAPTER 8: REAL SELF-CARE IS AN ASSERTION OF POWER: CLAIMING WHAT'S YOURS AND REMAKING THE SYSTEM

1. Arthur C. Brooks, "The Difference between Hope and Optimism," *Atlantic*, September 2019, theatlantic.com/family/archive/2021/09/hope-optimism-happiness /620164.

2. Fred B. Bryant et al., "Distinguishing Hope and Optimism: Two Sides of a Coin, or Two Separate Coins?" *Journal of Social and Clinical Psychology* 23, no. 2 (2004): 273–302.

3. Pooja Lakshmin et al., "Testimonial Psychotherapy in Immigrant Survivors of Intimate Partner Violence: A Case Series," *Transcultural Psychiatry* 55, no. 5 (October 2018): 585–600.

4. James L. Griffith, "Hope Modules: Brief Psychotherapeutic Interventions to Counter Demoralization from Daily Stressors of Chronic Illness," *Academic Psychiatry* 42, no. 1 (February 2018): 135–45.

5. Quote from Angela Garbes at Chamber of Mothers Summit, May 4, 2022.

6. Audre Lorde, commencement address at Oberlin College, 1989.

7. M. M. Varna et al., "Prosocial Behavior Promotes Positive Emotion during the COVID-19 Pandemic," *Emotion* (2022), psycnet.apa.org/fulltext/2022-42967 -001.html.